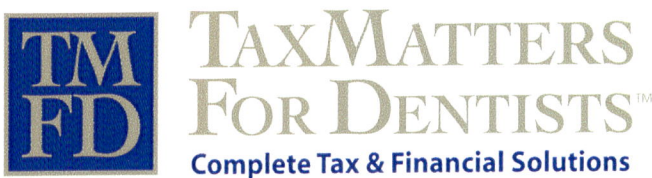

Align your practice with your life

350 Burnhamthorpe Rd. West
Suite 218, Mississauga, ON, L5B 3J1

Tel: 905-273-6605 • Fax: 905-273-9260
info@tmfd.ca • www.tmfd.ca

More Praise for *Secrets of The Wealthy Dentist*

A must-read for every dentist, *Secrets of the Wealthy Dentist* is a detailed road map to financial success no matter what stage of your career you find yourself in.

Dr. Neil Gajjar, DDS, MAGD, FADI, FPFA, FICD

Secrets of the Wealthy Dentist is a great guide for dentists of any age to follow in achieving financial success and retirement freedom.

Dr. Leny Sferlazza, DDS, MAGD, FICOI

This compelling story of three dentists reminds all of us in the dental profession that we're not alone. The financial challenges we face can't be handled in isolation. As this parable so vividly illustrates, there's no shame in seeking out a group of trusted advisors to help us through the maze of decisions that confront us.

Dr. Arthur Johnston, DDS

Secrets of the Wealthy Dentist offers true insight into the personal and professional management of a dentist's life. Having practiced dentistry for over 20 years, I've been through every step outlined in this book, except for the last transition into retirement. You'll be amazed at the excellent tax-saving strategies. After all, it's not how much you make that counts, but how much you save.

Dr. Jitendra Mistry, DMD

Every dentist who cares about their financial health should read this book. When it comes to financial planning, most of us procrastinate even though we know we shouldn't. This book helps demystify the planning process to give you the jump start you need. *Secrets of the Wealthy Dentist* takes into account that we're dentists, not accountants, by combining facts and numbers with a compelling story to create an easy and enjoyable read.

Dr. Murray Arlin, DDS, dip. Perio., F.R.C.D.(C)

You learned how to be an excellent dentist in dental school but not how to profitably run a practice or manage your finances. This book spells it all out. *Secrets of the Wealthy Dentist* is an easy-to-understand guide full of valuable financial planning strategies, tips and solutions.
Dr. Roger P. Levin, DDS
Chairman & CEO, Levin Group, Inc.

You're a dentist, not an accountant. This book spells out how to find a team specializing in your needs to coordinate your financial affairs, and the concrete benefits of doing so.
Ettore Palmeri, MBA, AGDM, BEd, BA
President, Palmeri Publishing Inc.

Secrets of the Wealthy Dentist describes three scenarios that a dentist could face while engaged in the practice of dentistry. Along the way, the book provides valuable hints and advice on financial matters that affect us all, both professionally and personally, and shows us how to keep more of the money we make. A highly recommended resource.
Dr. Pravin Patel, DDS

Secrets of the Wealthy Dentist is an insightful how-to guide written by experienced financial planners who understand dentists' needs and the opportunities they can too easily overlook.
Dan Sullivan
Founder, Strategic Coach Inc.

Great book... easy to read. I wish I had such a useful resource when I first graduated over 20 years ago. This book should be on the recommended list for all dentists in private practice as it would significantly facilitate their understanding of the business of dentistry.
Dr. Guido Galli, DDS, dip. Perio.

A Business Parable for Dental Professionals

SECRETS OF THE

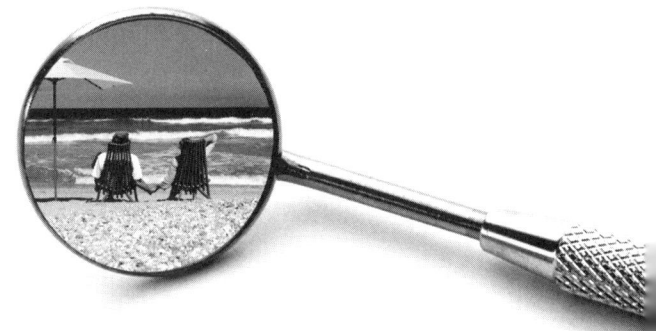

WEALTHY DENTIST

MIKE LAKHANI
With **STIVE FARRONATO** and **CHRIS MOLLOY**

© 2012 Tax Matters for Dentists

All rights reserved. No part of this book may be reproduced or transmitted in any form or by any means, electronic or mechanical, including photocopying, recording, or by any information storage and retrieval system without the prior written permission of the author, except for the inclusion of brief quotations in critical review and certain other non-commerial uses permitted by copyright law. For permission requests, contact the author in writing at the address below.

ISBN 978-0-9869337-0-7

Publisher's Cataloguing-in-Publication data

Library and Archives Canada Cataloguing in Publication
Lakhani, Mike, 1949-
Secrets of the wealthy dentist: a business parable for dental professionals / Mike Lakhani with Stive Farronato and Chris Molloy.
Issued also in an electronic format.

ISBN 978-0-9869337-0-7

1. Dentists—Finance, Personal. 2. Dentistry—Practice—Finance.
I. Farronato, Stive, 1966- II. Molloy, Chris, 1971-III. Title.

RK58.L35 2011   332.024'6176   C2011-904454-4

First Edition

Tax Matters for Dentists
218-350 Burnhamthorpe Road West
Mississauga, ON
L5B 3J1

Printed in Canada

Material in this book is for educational purposes only. This book is sold with the understanding that neither the author nor the publisher is rendering legal, accounting, tax, investment, or other professional services by publishing this book. This publication is not a substitute for the advice of your financial advisor or any of your other advisors, personal or professional.

*To all the dentists who have
worked with us over the years,
thank you for your trust.*

Contents

	Preface	ix
	Acknowledgements	xiii
Section I:	**Dr. Malhotra's Education**	1
	1. Three dentists	3
	2. A chance meeting	9
	3. The Good Samaritan	17
	4. Advice acted on	19
	5. The appointment	23
	6. His life on paper	37
	7. Incorporation	41
	8. New beginnings	49
	9. Tweaking the plan	59
	Financial Profile: Dr. Malhotra	65

Section II:	**Dr. Bekker's Struggles**	71
	10. A step in the right direction	73
	11. Eyes wide open	81
	12. Changing course	85
	13. The numbers	93
	14. Ready for change	99
	15. Passing the budget	103
	16. What they decided	113
	17. Giving thanks for good advice	117
	Financial Profile: Dr. Bekker	119
Section III:	**Dr. St. Louis' Exit Strategy**	127
	18. Planning for retirement	129
	19. Smart investments	133
	20. Security within reach	143
	21. The exit strategy	145
	22. The defining issue: a share- or asset-based sale	149
	23. The final stretch	153
	24. Celebrating with friends	159
	Financial Profile: Dr. St. Louis	165
	Epilogue	173
	About the Authors	175

Preface

The idea for this book was developed after years of publishing my newsletter, *Tax Matters for Dentists*. Together with my partners and co-authors, Stive Farronato and Chris Molloy, I write case studies about actual client scenarios and the solutions provided to improve their situations. After creating a collection of case studies, I wanted to expand upon these concepts and explore them in detail. More importantly, I wanted to demonstrate the benefits these changes could have on clients' lifestyles once aligned with their main source of revenue—their dental practices.

The Format

In developing this book's format, I asked myself how I could introduce tax and financial planning concepts in an engaging and interesting way. As I've said many times in my seminars, my objective isn't to make accountants out of dentists!

I decided to create a story about three characters, at various stages in their careers, whose paths cross in their quest to find coordinated solutions to their financial concerns. I used a parable format so the reader could better identify with the financial challenges faced by the story's characters. As a dentist reading this book, you may come to recognize you aren't alone in your concerns and challenges.

The Numbers

In this book, I describe various financial planning concepts. I've always found that actual numbers illustrate the impact of these concepts far better than words alone, which is why there's a summary of calculations supporting each section. I hope the summaries will satisfy those readers who want to know the mechanics behind the calculations. Those who'd rather not be bothered with the details can pass over these sections without compromising the messages in the story.

The Principles

My experience has repeatedly shown that most dentists use advisors in isolation, specifically for one purpose at a time—banks for practice financing, consultants for practice management, stockbrokers for investments, insurance agents for risk management, lawyers for estate planning, and accountants for tax preparation. While all these functions are necessary, the dentist is often left to coordinate the activities and liaise between each party. The time, effort, and potential miscommunication can be costly or exhausting. Using the services of a trusted advisor to coordinate the duties of these various experts, however, can result in significant cash flow improvement and much less stress for the dental practitioner.

This book contains many of my fundamental financial planning beliefs about tax reduction, efficient cash flow management, and building net worth. A key principle is that the incorporation of a dental practice can be beneficial in a vast majority of situations. In the short term, incorporation offers the opportunity for tax savings and improved cash flow. In the long term, it offers efficient accumulation of investments for retirement, education funding for family members, structure for business succession, and estate planning opportunities.

Besides tax reduction strategies, investments are an important part of building net worth. While most often talked about at dinner parties or with colleagues, investing continues to be a widely misunderstood endeavour, characterized by irrational decisions and inappropriate risks. Emotion, non-stop media noise, and claims citing the ability to beat markets are huge distractions to investors. Sticking to a well-structured and personalized investment policy that addresses global diversification, risk management, tax allocation, and a low-cost index–based approach goes a long way in building net worth.

Align Your Practice with Your Life

As a dentist, your practice is the engine of wealth creation. Your practice needs to be integrated with your personal objectives to ensure you achieve your goals in the most effective way possible. The growth of your net worth is the benchmark that provides both the measure of your progress and a sense of comfort.

While there's no shortage of "great ideas" within the realm of personal finance, those ideas don't achieve much until they're actually implemented. I hope this story will motivate you to be proactive about achieving your personal financial objectives.

The key is to work with an advisor you can trust to coordinate with other professionals in managing your cash flow, taxes, and building your net worth. Ultimately, this will help you align your practice with your life.

Mike Lakhani
November 2011

Note: The tax planning techniques and tax rates used in this book are based on the rules in the province of Ontario in 2011. For simplicity, rounding has been used in some instances.

Acknowledgements

We would like to acknowledge many of the people who have guided us during our emergence into the dental industry.

Dr. Neil Gajjar was instrumental in introducing us to many members of the Ontario Academy of General Dentistry, OAGD, and to the various societies and study clubs in Ontario. As a result of his confidence in our team, he invited us to become one of the original sponsors of the South Asian Dental Association (SADA), to which we continue to provide support and offer speaking engagements at their events.

The success of our newsletter, *Tax Matters for Dentists*, couldn't have been accomplished without the services of Ettore Palmeri, of Palmeri Publishing Inc. Ettore graciously allowed our publication to be circulated with issues of *Spectrum Dialogue* and *Teamwork* magazines. This provided us with visibility to dental practitioners that we wouldn't have attained without his help.

We would also like to thank Rudi Rodrigues for his collaboration with Ettore in the creative elements, layout, and design of the newsletter.

Aside from the publication, we have gained greater exposure to dentists in the Greater Toronto Area through our speaking engagements. We would again like to thank Ettore Palmeri, principal of the Aethestic Design & Implant Academy (formerly Toronto Implant and Aesthetic Study Club), and founder Dr. Murray Arlin for allowing us the opportunity to present at their events many times over the years.

Our success truly is a reflection of a team effort. We would also like to thank our staff and family members who have supported us behind the scenes. Without their continued dedication to our efforts, this book and our success within the dental community wouldn't be possible.

Section I: Dr. Malhotra's Education

Chapter 1: Three dentists

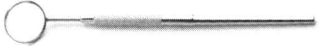

Dr. Malhotra: 7:00 a.m.
On the first morning of the Ontario Dental Association (ODA) annual spring meeting, traffic was congested and frustrating to navigate in and around Toronto. By city standards, that meant the crawl of traffic was frequently slowing to a complete halt. Dr. Arjun Malhotra lived in London, Ontario, so he wasn't used to it at all. It was nothing like London traffic. But being a patient man, Dr. Malhotra kept his wits about him and kept his mind occupied with the latest book on tape he'd borrowed from the library. His long commutes to work during the week were often boring; the audio tapes kept his mind occupied, and it was the only way possible to get through some of the books he wanted to read for pleasure.

He hadn't driven in Toronto in at least four months, and then it was only to pick up a cousin at the airport on the outskirts of the city. His drives to work were often white-knuckle stuff in the winter, but all that snow and ice paled in comparison to the madness of downtown Toronto traffic. *How do Torontonians do it?* Dr. Malhotra wondered.

The first hour of the drive into Toronto was easy enough—that part was familiar to him as he'd been commuting for the past eighteen months to an office in Kitchener where he worked as an associate two days a week. He'd practically worn grooves into the asphalt along the route between his hometown of London and Kitchener. He could name the exits by heart. Between those drives and the forty-minute, once-a-week commutes he made out to Strathroy to work as an associate at a practice in town, Dr. Malhotra was running his four-year-old Volkswagen Golf into the ground.

By the time he reached Mississauga, his clock was moving faster than his odometer. He still had a good hour to go before he'd be anywhere near the city centre. A thick fog had rolled in and caused a couple of fender-benders on the 401, which had basically shut down the highway. Nobody was moving an inch. Dr. Malhotra thought that perhaps he should have brought another book on tape. What he was certain of was that he was running more than an hour late—and it wasn't his nature to be late.

He was eager to make it to the conference. It was his second year attending, and if the previous year was any indication, this year would prove to be very informative. He was looking forward to the sessions on cosmetic dentistry. He also had plans to meet a couple of old classmates for breakfast. He hadn't seen Thom and Darcy since they had all graduated from the University of Western Ontario two years before. It was hard to get together often because none of them lived in the same city, so the meeting was a good opportunity to catch up—other than in brief and sporadic e-mails. They were bound to hassle him because he still drove the same car he'd had in university, especially since Darcy had recently purchased a gorgeous black Mercedes.

The upside to traffic congestion was that the delay was sparing him those shots. The way it was working out, he'd be lucky to get a coffee to go at the convention centre before the opening session.

Dr. Bekker 7:25 a.m.
Dr. Dennis Bekker was only coming from Bayview and Lawrence and should have been able to make it to the conference on time, but as luck would have it, Dr. Bekker was sitting in his vermilion red BMW M3, noticing that the "check engine" light was on again. He'd first discovered this on the drive back from his cottage in Muskoka the previous Sunday night. Trish, his eternally optimistic wife, assured him that it hadn't been on the last time she'd driven the car. It really annoyed him because there were less than thirty thousand clicks on the vehicle. Then again, he had no idea what went on with the BMW when the kids borrowed the car. He trusted them to share any major information, but small hiccups in the car's performance might not be something they'd want to admit to for fear of not being allowed to use it again. Why he even let them use the BMW, he wasn't sure. He'd thought many times about getting them a Kia or some compact economy car for them to ride around in, but it never went much past the idea stage. He'd have to get the vehicle to the mechanic sometime this week.

The BMW's GPS showed that there were eleven kilometres to the Metro Toronto Convention Centre, which would take about seventeen minutes on a good day. Like Dr. Malhotra, Dr. Bekker had colleagues he wanted to catch up with; if nothing else, it'd be good to get a laugh from Dr. Manser's receding hairline. Even though their school days were long behind them, they'd stayed in touch over the years by e-mail, but nothing replaced face-to-face conversations. But this morning, real life was getting in the way. He'd dropped off the twins at riding school down by Sunnybrook earlier in the morning and was now shuffling them across Lawrence Avenue to Havergal College. "It'd be nice if you girls could ride over to school," Dr. Bekker laughed. He looked in the rearview mirror and saw Tracey and Anna rolling their eyes at him. Another reminder of just how uncool they thought he was.

Finally, he dropped the twins off at school at 7:45 a.m. and made his way downtown to the meeting. His stomach was growling and he thought he might stop at McDonald's, but the GPS wasn't equipped to indicate how long the lineups at the drive-through windows would last, so he'd have to grab a quick bite and go straight into the conference hall.

Dr. St. Louis 7:45 a.m.

At quarter to eight, the food court at the convention centre was close to capacity. Dr. Adeline St. Louis had been one of the first to sit down. She'd flown in the night before from Ottawa and had already filed away her breakfast receipt in the small file folder she carried in her large Coach bag. Always an early riser, Dr. St. Louis had asked for a 6 a.m. wake-up call and made her way to the gym for a forty-five-minute walk on the treadmill, a quick steam in the sauna, and then a shower.

At the table in the restaurant, Dr. St. Louis pored through the *Globe and Mail* and gave the "Report on Business" a close reading over a breakfast of yogurt and cereal. She'd also brought along a good book—her husband always insisted on having two with him whenever he traveled, even if it was just a commute across town. He'd happily forget his wallet before he forgot something to read. "Never know when you'll have to wait for a tow truck," he'd say.

She teased him about it—"a hopeless academic who'd seek shelter from a storm in a book." Tucked away in a side pocket was the latest from Scott Turow, a slight departure from her usual choice of story, but a hygienist in her office had highly recommended it. After twenty-five years of marriage, Dr. St. Louis and her husband had picked up each other's habits (and the book habit had served her well the time a two-hour stopover at Heathrow became an eight-hour ordeal).

By 7:50 a.m. her reading had slowed down considerably, her progress interrupted frequently by visits from peers, friends, and those who'd sat on committees she chaired, which were quite a few, as Dr. St. Louis had been a member of the association for almost thirty years. She wondered whether she would still be interested in attending these conferences once she finally retired from dentistry. Retirement wasn't far off, and she was already making mental notes about the travel plans she and her husband wished to pursue.

When the tide of people eventually trickled to a halt, she put her book aside and checked the weather in New York on her iPhone. She and her husband had tickets to a couple of Broadway shows the following weekend.

Chapter 2: A chance meeting

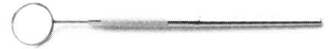

At 8:00 a.m., half an hour before the meeting's scheduled start, word circulated that it was delayed by forty-five minutes and would now start at 9:15 a.m. Dr. St. Louis overheard the news; it was confirmed by a colleague's text message. Apparently, there were problems with the wireless microphones and recording devices in the seminar rooms, so the morning presentations had to be delayed until the equipment was fixed.

At 8:05 a.m., Dr. Malhotra pulled the Golf into a parking lot off of Front Street and found a spot reserved for compact cars. Meanwhile, Dr. Bekker was finding traffic so snarled that he didn't even try to get down to the south building of the Convention Centre, where the conference was being held. He gave up his hunt for a spot on the street and turned into the first public parking lot he could find on Queen St. He broke into a breathless run, jaywalking and weaving between cars like a halfback following his blockers. By the time he reached Front Street, he found himself standing next to Dr. Malhotra. They glanced at each other. Dr. Bekker noticed the younger dentist wearing a lanyard and a name tag.

"Are you on your way to the ODA meeting?" Dr. Bekker asked Dr. Malhotra.

"I am. Finally found parking." Dr. Malhotra looked at his watch. "We don't have much time, do we?"

"No. Traffic was horrible and of course finding a spot was maddening. I'll have to buy a coffee to take in with me. No time for a sit-down meal this morning. There's a pretty decent food court, marché style, at the Convention Centre." Dr. Bekker pulled out his phone and opened a text message. "Oh, hey, one of my colleagues just informed me that the meeting's been delayed to 9:15 a.m. Looks like time is suddenly on our side. I'm Dr. Dennis Bekker. And you are. . .?"

"Dr. Arjun Malhotra."

Dr. Bekker and Dr. Malhotra made their way to the convention centre, stopping to ask the doorman for directions to the food court because they now had time to eat a proper meal. By the time they found it, the place was full; other dentists had retreated there to wait out the delay with a better breakfast than just muffins. The only two unoccupied seats were at Dr. St. Louis' table beside the window. Dr. Malhotra nervously asked Dr. St. Louis if she was alone and if she would mind if he and Dr. Bekker joined her.

"Please. I've been sitting here quite a while, so some company is absolutely welcome," she said.

The three exchanged introductions.

"Where do you both practise?" Dr. St. Louis asked.

"I'm an associate at offices in London, Kitchener, and Strathroy. This is my second ODA meeting. I think it'll be a great opportunity to network and talk to colleagues who are much more experienced," said Dr. Malhotra somewhat sheepishly. He was keenly aware of the age difference between the three of them, and he was feeling less confident than he'd anticipated.

"I have a practice here in the city, going on twenty years now. Been to so many of these association meetings, but I haven't attended in years. Family life prevents me from making it a lot of the time. I'll have three kids over eighteen soon anyway, so it gets nuts sometimes. I missed last year's conference because of a week-long trip to Paris. But I do enjoy them because it's a great way to catch up and meet new colleagues like you," Dr. Bekker said.

Dr. Malhotra excused himself for a moment while he went to buy some oatmeal. Dr. Bekker, hungrier than he thought, went off to a creperie counter. He hadn't had a crepe in ages—double ham and cheese was what he craved. Maybe even chocolate banana.

When Dr. Malhotra returned with his cereal, Dr. St. Louis made small talk; she could tell that the young dentist felt uncomfortable.

"Did you grow up in London?" she asked.

"My family came to Canada when I was three. I was born in Delhi. My younger brother was born here, though."

"My husband and I were in Delhi last year," Dr. St. Louis said, delighted they had a point of interest they could share. "We toured extensively in the north of the subcontinent, but Delhi was one of our most spectacular stops. We were amazed by the Red Fort and the Jantar Mantar . . . who could have imagined such an incredible observatory built in the eighteenth century?"

Dr. Bekker returned to the table with his crepes. He hadn't heard Dr. St. Louis talking about her experiences in Delhi.

"What took you to India?" Dr. Malhotra asked.

"My husband is a professor of classics, so we had an extended summer," she told him. "Some summers he has research that he undertakes abroad, and I can have some younger associates step in for me for longer than my usual vacation time."

"It's great that you can travel like that," Dr. Malhotra said. "I feel like I'm running as fast as I can just to keep up. I can't seem to get ahead. Two years out of school, and I'm still paying down my student loans. I'm trying to help out my parents, but I feel like I can't do enough. I took a couple of weeks off and went to a friend's cottage for a long weekend, but otherwise I didn't get away this year. I always imagined that it'd be easier than this. I knew it wouldn't be possible to have overnight success, but this amount of time wasn't what I expected at all."

Dr. St. Louis nodded and smiled sympathetically. Dr. Malhotra was fishing for advice, and she knew that.

"It wasn't a matter of me being a financial whiz," Dr. St. Louis said. "I can assure you I'm not. It was hard for me, too, coming out of dental school. It was hard for quite a few years beyond that, even. It was only when my husband and I went to the Leighton team that things got better."

"

If you don't have a plan and if you don't have help, you can spend years working hard but not achieve your financial potential.

"

Dr. Malhotra looked confused, so she added, "They're tax advisors to dentists. I know, I hardly would've thought such a thing existed but it does, and I'm so thankful for it. I'd always thought that if I worked hard enough, things would look after themselves. And I'd always been independent—asking someone else for help wasn't something I was comfortable doing.

"The truth is that if you don't have a plan and if you don't have help, you can spend years working hard but not achieve your financial potential. But because we had a plan and stayed with it over the years, we saw a big difference from one year to the next."

Dr. Malhotra asked Dr. St. Louis how long ago she'd first solicited advice from the Leighton team. She did the math.

"How time flies. More than fifteen years ago now. I graduated from McGill over thirty years ago," she said, "but in many ways I did my graduate studies when I met the Leighton team and learned about the business of my practice—what I should've been doing from day one."

Dr. Malhotra's eyebrows arched. "It wasn't just a one-time deal where they helped organize your practice?" he asked.

"No. We've developed a relationship over the years," Dr. St. Louis said. "They've helped me look beyond the numbers, to focus on the long-term objectives of my husband and myself."

Dr. Malhotra hadn't been the most materialistic in his circle of friends during university, and his family had always stressed the idea of living modestly. Nevertheless, he couldn't help but notice Dr. St. Louis' watch. He didn't know much about watches, but he knew Chanel was a top name and was certain hers was worth more than his car.

"I wish I could be doing half as well as you are," Dr. Malhotra said, instantly regretting the admission the minute the words came out of his mouth. There was no envy, just a wish that his hard work in school and in his first years of practice had been as rewarding as he'd expected when he chose to pursue dentistry as a career. Dr. St. Louis' response surprised him.

"Well, I wish I were starting today like you are and had a chance to realize the benefits of a well-managed practice. One of the best pieces of advice I received from the Leighton team early on was the importance of focusing on my dental practice and not other ventures. Nothing else comes close for generating cash flow for the future." Dr. St. Louis thought again about her plans to retire in a couple of years and sell her practice. She hadn't let some of her long-time friends know that the Leighton team was already working on it for her. It was best not to bring the matter up until all the *i*'s had been dotted and the *t*'s had been crossed. She opened her Day-Timer, pulled out a business card, and handed it to Dr. Malhotra. "Call or e-mail me if you want to know more," she said.

> *One of the best pieces of advice I received early on was the importance of focusing on my dental practice and not other ventures. Nothing else comes close for generating cash flow for the future.*

"Thank you, Dr. St. Louis. I don't have a card to give you in return."

"I'll get your contact info once you e-mail me. And, please, call me Adeline."

Dr. Bekker's breakfast had his undivided attention. He still had part of his breakfast left when his cell phone vibrated. He looked at the call display: his son calling from Queen's University. He knew what was going to follow—another plea for cash. Dr. Bekker felt the urge to let the call go to voice mail but felt too guilty.

"Yes, Clayton, what's going on? I'm in a bit of a rush."

"Dad, my laptop died on me. I think it's the logic board. The guy at the Apple shop says it's going to cost a fortune to fix. Can you help me out? I have four papers to hand in next week, and I'm totally up the creek without my files."

Dr. Bekker sighed. "Okay, Clay. I'll go to the bank later today and transfer money to your account. Find out first how much to get it fixed. Don't buy anything new or added or extra. I gotta go, kid. Don't worry, it's all going to be just fine." He hung up and gulped a large amount of coffee before it went cold.

When Dr. Malhotra and Dr. St. Louis looked over, Dr. Bekker rolled his eyes. "Kids. Can't live without them but can't afford them, either. If it isn't someone's Mac dying, it's some repair my wife wants done or school trips for the twins." Dr. Bekker felt like it was all piling up. On the drive to the conference, he'd received a text reminder from his wife: *contractor coming by at dinnertime . . . marble counter . . . bathroom?* Sometimes, when things actually fell into place, he felt eminently qualified to be a dentist *and* an air-traffic controller. Or maybe a fireman, because it seemed all he did away from the office was put out one fire after another (with occasional breaks for golf).

Dr. St. Louis passed a business card to Dr. Bekker. "E-mail me and I'll send you the same information I'm sending Arjun about the Leighton team. I think they could really help you. It's worth investigating, at any rate."

At that point, it was ten after nine and the meeting was about to begin. The three dentists bade farewell to one another and headed off to the meeting hall, pleased to have expanded their network of colleagues. Dr. Malhotra was doubly pleased because he'd discovered that maybe all wasn't lost and that he could have a bright future sooner than he was beginning to think.

Chapter 3: The Good Samaritan

The three dentists moved in their own circles that day. During the breaks, Dr. St. Louis caught up with dentists who, like her, would have struggled to count how many of these meetings they'd attended over their long careers. A couple she'd met at the previous year's meeting thanked her for recommending the Leighton team. The advice they had received had brought peace and stability to their lives.

On the other side of the conference hall, Dr. Bekker chatted with friends who also had well-established, lucrative practices in downtown Toronto, as well as sons and daughters in university or heading there in the next couple of years. Over lunch, Dr. Malhotra compared notes with Mike, a former roommate from school days, and had managed to meet up with his college friends for a coffee in the cappuccino lounge. And, as he'd predicted, Mike had made a jab about the old Volkswagen.

After the final educational track for the day, Dr. Malhotra jumped into his Golf to head uptown. Mike had told him about a sale at Harry Rosen, and Dr. Malhotra wanted to pick something up—maybe a nice silk tie or shirt—for himself and his father, whose birthday was coming up. Dr. Malhotra saw a man standing in front of a car with the hood open, pleading with a parking attendant. When Dr. Malhotra slowed down, he recognized the distressed driver as Dr. Bekker. Dr. Malhotra pulled over and asked Dr. Bekker what was wrong.

"It won't turn over," Dr. Bekker said. "Something's been wrong with this heap for the last few days. The red engine light kept coming on. I don't know why I shouldn't scrap it completely."

"Try to start the car again."

Dr. Bekker did, and then when nothing happened, he threw Dr. Malhotra a look that said *See?* The battery was almost flat.

"Let me get my cables and give you a boost. I can follow you to a garage."

"You keep cables with you?" Dr. Bekker asked, impressed. Dr. Malhotra was nothing if not practical. Dr. Bekker bought provisional items like that but never had them on hand when he actually needed them. He'd bought some contraption that inflated a tire on the roadside, but the day he'd had a flat on the 401, it was somewhere in the family's garage. His wife reminded him of it whenever they passed someone with a flat tire.

"All the winter driving I do getting to the offices I'm an associate at," Dr. Malhotra said, "I need to have these things. I do have CAA insurance, but you never know how long they'll take to get to you. Always a good idea to have them on hand."

Dr. Bekker deeply appreciated Dr. Malhotra's assistance. "When you're in Toronto next time, give me a call," he said. "Taking you to lunch is the least I can do for all of this."

Chapter 4: Advice acted on

One night a week later, Dr. Malhotra was at home, sitting in front of his computer screen. He'd e-mailed his younger brother Ramesh to see if he was still on track for the scholarship money he'd been awarded. Then he uploaded some recent family photos to his Facebook account; a cousin in Delhi had asked to see them. He also sent him a message that said, *It's been so long since I've seen you . . . I wish I were there.* Dr. Malhotra pushed the keyboard away; his mind was racing. *I wish I could do more for my brother.*

Dr. Malhotra had received some scholarship money, but it had offered only partial financial relief, and he knew it'd be the same for his brother. The first lesson of university life is the high price of hidden and miscellaneous costs. *I wish I could see my cousin and his family*, thought Dr. Malhotra. He could either go to Delhi or help them come here for a visit—it didn't matter much. But it'd be a major expense, and wasn't something he could do right now.

There were too many other things he had to do financially first. Dr. Malhotra pushed the keyboard away and leaned back in his chair. *It should be easier.*

Dr. Malhotra thought about Dr. St. Louis and the lifestyle she and her husband enjoyed—it was the lifestyle he'd been working toward in dental school. He didn't feel that his life lacked any rewards, but he hadn't received the rewards he'd expected, such as being able to travel.

Rifling through his Day-Timer, he found the business card Dr. St. Louis had given him. He started a new e-mail:

> *Dr. St. Louis,*
> *I'm the young dentist who talked with you at breakfast before the conference the other day. You mentioned a group that gives you financial advice in operating your practice. Could you provide me with the contact information? It would be deeply appreciated.*
> *Hope you and your husband are doing well.*
>
> *Many thanks,*
> *Dr. Arjun Malhotra*

When Dr. Malhotra checked his e-mail a few hours later, he had a reply from Dr. St. Louis.

> *Arjun,*
> *It was great to meet you at the conference. My husband and I are doing quite well. We had a wonderful weekend in New York, and we're looking at something a little more adventurous for our anniversary weekend—Paris, if I have my way.*

You'll find the contact information for the Leighton team below. Please feel free to use my name as a reference when you give them a call. I'm sure you'll find the group very helpful. I know I do.

Best Wishes,
Adeline

Chapter 5: The appointment

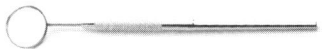

The day after receiving the information from Dr. St. Louis, Dr. Malhotra called up the Leighton office to arrange an appointment to meet with someone. Two weeks later, after a full morning of appointments in Kitchener, Dr. Malhotra drove to Mississauga for a meeting with Paul Leighton, senior advisor at the Leighton team. He brought the file full of financial documents with him that had been requested at the time he set up the appointment.

The meeting made him more uncomfortable than excited. He'd mentioned it to one of the hygienists at the Kitchener practice. "It's like my trip to the dentist," Dr. Malhotra had said. The joke had gotten a laugh from her, but Dr. Malhotra had been telling the truth. When he sat down with Paul Leighton in the company's offices, it was the closest thing he'd experienced to white-jacket syndrome. The idea of reviewing his finances made him nervous, and in the days before the meeting he'd seriously considered rescheduling and even dropping the whole thing.

Dr. Malhotra was once again thinking about abandoning the idea as he started completing the confidential questionnaire he'd been given to fill out while he waited for Paul Leighton. The form was a standard piece of paperwork that clients prepare for financial planners. But even the overview page left Dr. Malhotra puzzled. For instance, he had no idea what "planning assumptions" meant, nor had he given much thought to the rate of inflation, never mind making any assumptions about it. Furthermore, retirement seemed so far off that he didn't know where to start with the line that read *Retirement needs (annually, in today's dollar, indexed to inflation)—after tax*. And he had no idea where to start with the line under that one: *Survivor's Needs (%)*.

Dr. Malhotra didn't have any survivor candidates in mind, so projecting the needs of a future bride (or the needs of the family they'd raise) seemed like too much blue-sky imagining, like putting the cart before the horse. His energy right now was directed toward working full-time and paying down his student debt. He hadn't thought about when he'd like to retire or whether his financial needs would increase or decrease over the term of his retirement.

It was then that Paul Leighton popped his head out from his office. He walked over to Dr. Malhotra, extending his hand. "Good to meet you, Dr. Malhotra. I'm Paul Leighton. How are you making out with those forms?"

"Mr. Leighton—"

"Please, call me Paul. No need for formality. Over the next few months, I'm going to know everything there is to know about you, so we may as well be on a first-name basis, don't you think?"

Dr. Malhotra nodded. "The forms are very involved. I hadn't expected them to be so detailed. I'm not even done reviewing them. Sorry."

SECTION I: DR. MALHOTRA'S EDUCATION

"Absolutely no need to apologize, Arjun. Please come into my office and finish up in there. I have some things to discuss with my receptionist anyway. I'll check in on you in five minutes." Paul left, closing the door behind him, and Dr. Malhotra resumed reviewing the forms.

SIN and *Birthdate* he could fill in, but *Life Expectancy*? How was he supposed to project that? The projections sections weren't the only parts that had slowed him down—the here-and-now sections were also trouble. He didn't have a name to write in beside *Investment Advisor* or *Life Insurance Agent*. His parents had nagged him a little about getting life insurance, but he didn't have a clue about what was involved and certainly didn't have the time to figure it out. He felt sheepish circling *No* beside *Wills prepared?* and *Powers of Attorney? Education fund*? That seemed ridiculously premature, and not just because he wasn't married yet and didn't have any children—he was still paying off his own student loan.

In the end, Dr. Malhotra felt like he'd only half-filled out the form because he'd slashed out or left blank so many sections. The more pages he'd flipped through and marked only lightly, the more he felt like he'd walked into an unfamiliar room, with the lights off, and had to go in search of a paper clip or thumbtack. The proverbial needle in the haystack.

Paul re-entered his office and sat at his desk, across from Dr. Malhotra.

"How did the last parts go? You'd be surprised by how many people actually find this part very difficult and rather disconcerting, so know that you're not the first, nor will you be the last."

In the short time that his patients had been seeing Dr. Malhotra, most thought highly of him because of his good work and chair-side manner. His soft-spoken manner and meticulous attention put all but the chronically jittery at ease. For a young dentist, he was unusually accomplished in the social aspect of his job, and it was in much the same way that Paul Leighton managed to put him at ease.

"Well, I did what I could. . . ." Dr. Malhotra pulled out his somewhat-completed questionnaire and opened his file containing the other documents he'd been asked to bring. He laid them on the table and planned on going through explanations, document by document, line by line. He was about to stand up to get a better view of the numbers when Paul raised his hand. Paul had seen this sort of thing many times before and gently motioned to Dr. Malhotra to sit down.

"I'm interested in the numbers, Arjun, but let's set them aside for a moment," Paul said. "Start by telling me about yourself, not about your professional life, but about your personal life."

"My life story?" Dr. Malhotra hadn't come prepared for this!

"If you want to put it that way, sure."

Dr. Malhotra paused. *Where to start?* It wasn't something that he was used to doing—patients who came in for an examination or dental work never asked him for his life story, just an assessment. He noticed a picture of Paul and his wife and family on the wall. And he noticed a framed photo of Paul with his family standing somewhere obviously warm, with palm trees in the background. He sighed, knowing these were things he wanted, as well, but simply had no idea how to achieve them.

Over the next twenty minutes, Dr. Malhotra talked about his life and his family. He explained how he'd been born in Delhi but had come to Canada when he was young and moved to London in elementary school. He told Paul how his father had started out with a job on the floor of a factory, had worked his way up to foreman ten years later, and was now looking forward to retirement, hopefully before he reached his mid-sixties. He explained how his mother stayed at home—she'd worked in child care, but a back injury made it difficult for her to work more than a couple of short shifts a week. And then there was his brother, who hoped to follow in his footsteps to university, perhaps studying something in the sciences, maybe dentistry, or maybe medicine. He also mentioned his extended family in Delhi and how he wished he could see them more.

"Good. That gives me a better idea as to where you're coming from. Now I need to know some details about you."

Dr. Malhotra was never comfortable with being the centre of attention, and he was even less comfortable talking about himself; it was easier to speak about the family of which he was so proud.

"What exactly do you want to know about me?" he asked Paul.

"Well, let's start with the basics. How old are you?"

"Thirty last month."

"Where did you go to school?"

"The Schulich School at the University of Western Ontario."

"When did you graduate?"

"Two years ago."

"Are you married?"

"No, I'm single. But I hope to marry one day."

"In a relationship?"

Dr. Malhotra laughed. "Not right now. I honestly don't have the time, and I'd like to find the right girl so that at some point, we get married and have kids. But that's in the long term. The way work has been going for these first couple of years of my career . . . well, I don't have much energy for getting out there after work and socializing."

Paul made a few notes in his notebook and took many mental notes.

"What do you like to do?"

Dr. Malhotra looked puzzled, so Paul was more specific.

"How do you like to spend your time away from work? Do you have any hobbies or interests? Many of our clients are golfers," Paul said. "Some like to collect and restore cars, or have other hobbies they've taken up."

"Maybe it'll sound strange," Dr. Malhotra said, taking a breath, "but I don't golf . . . I just drive one, a four-year-old Golf that'll get me home if I'm lucky." Paul didn't bother to stifle a laugh. Dr. Malhotra looked at the photo of Paul and his family enjoying a vacation together and continued.

"I've never really wanted a sports car or a Hummer or something like that. It just wouldn't suit my needs. I don't have any expensive hobbies. I play some recreational cricket, and our team tours for matches on weekends every summer. The one thing that I'm passionate about, though, is food. I'm a foodie, whether it's going to very good restaurants or preparing meals. I think it's a carry-over from school days. There was a copy of *The Joy of Cooking* left behind at our fraternity house. Maybe it was a sign. My fraternity brothers made mac and cheese, and I was preparing a brisket. Nowadays, if I go out for a great meal, the next week I'm in my kitchen trying to make the same dish."

Paul laughed. "And I thought I was doing well to make pancakes for my kids Saturday morning," he said. "What about vacations and travel? Do you travel at all? Would you like to?"

Dr. Malhotra was almost too embarrassed to mention his "staycation" the previous summer. "No, not yet, but I want to start saving to take my parents and brother back to Delhi to see our relatives. It's been a long time, and our relatives back home could never afford to come here."

They spoke for another fifteen minutes. Talking about his life and family put Dr. Malhotra at ease. Paul gathered information that would give him a fuller picture than a ledger full of numbers would.

"Arjun, at the Leighton team we like to know our clients," he said. "We can do our best job for our clients when we know them well and develop a relationship over time. We want to have a good idea of our clients' needs and desires and want to know what the costs of supporting their lifestyle will be. I can tell from talking with you that you're quite conservative in your approach."

"That's one of the lessons of my childhood, I guess," Dr. Malhotra said. "It was difficult for us when we first came to Canada—I didn't realize it at the time, only later, but my parents worked very hard and they were conservative in the way they approached things. 'Be responsible' was the message that was driven home when I was growing up, the constant drumbeat."

"Well, I'm sure they're very proud of you and consider you a model son," Paul said. "And really, your decision to come here today isn't a high-risk proposition. It's really more a matter of reducing risks and positioning yourself for success."

"And that's a good thing," Dr. Malhotra said.

"Exactly," Paul said. "Now tell me about your life as an associate."

Dr. Malhotra laid out the basics: two days a week in London, two days in Kitchener, and one in Strathroy, working alongside established dentists. "In a good week, that's six hours of commuting," Dr. Malhotra said. "And in the winter, who knows? I'm improving my technical skills all the time, and I'm looking forward to the day I can set up my own office in London."

"Well, that's definitely something we can help you with and get you on the right track," Paul said. "We have strategies on structuring financing for the purchase of a practice, and the negotiations with the banks are something we can handle for you. We'll find the best possible rate."

Dr. Malhotra's mind raced. Purchasing a practice had been something he imagined he'd do in a few years once he felt his skills and confidence had improved. What had seemed like a matter for the far-off future suddenly sounded possible—maybe not tomorrow, but something that he wouldn't have to wait ten years to do.

Paul sipped his coffee and set down the cup. "Do you want some coffee?"

"No, thanks. I'm nervous enough as it is."

"No need to be. This is the first step in the right direction. Well, I feel like I know more about you than when we set this meeting up, so it's only fair that you know more about me and what we do here," Paul said.

Dr. Malhotra slipped back into his seat.

"I went to school in England and did my accounting degree there."

Dr. Malhotra had seen the paperwork on the wall of the office but hadn't looked closely enough to notice the school that had issued it.

"I met my wife there. We came to Canada from the UK over twenty-five years ago. For a time I ran a small business—a shop that built space heaters. I didn't imagine I was really destined to do that for my career, but I think it gave me an important background. As an accountant, you're trained to look at balance sheets, assess the numbers, and come up with strategies, but you can only really appreciate business, especially a small business, if you've actually had to do it yourself. Not dentistry per se, but there are common elements to all businesses."

It was something that Dr. Malhotra had thought about before, especially when discussing plans for his own practice with his parents. "My father always worked for the company. Even when he worked his way up in the company, it was supervision on the factory floor, not ownership. My father knew there was nothing quite like owning your own business, and it's what he wants for me. I know I'll have to be responsible for managing staff and ensuring the highest standard of care for my patients. I'll need to maintain education credits and stay on top of the latest industry regulations, and there's probably a host of other things I haven't considered yet," Dr. Malhotra said.

"

Some amendments and changes to provincial regulations in recent years have offered dentists some tax relief through incorporation and a chance to fare much better.

"

"Your father's a smart man, and you're right—there's a lot to consider before starting your own business, or practice in your case. Now, where was I? Oh yes. I managed to sell that business and moved back into accounting and financial planning," Paul said. "And I ended up working with a variety of clients, and among them were several dentists. Some of them, Dr. St. Louis for one, I've worked with for over fifteen years now. I'll admit, when I was in university, I didn't envision working with dentists as part of *my* practice. It just sort of evolved. But it was in working closely with these clients that we realized there were opportunities for them that their peers didn't realize. We also understood that there were aspects of tax law that worked against their interests."

Dr. Malhotra didn't like the sound of that. *Against their interests* made it sound like a brick wall that he'd be pushing up against.

"But some amendments and changes to provincial regulations in recent years have offered dentists some tax relief through incorporation and a chance to fare much better. And that's how our group has attracted so many dentists as clients. Over time, we've come to understand the demands of their practices and the opportunities too many of their peers miss."

Dr. Malhotra sighed, relieved to hear there wouldn't be a brick wall after all.

"We've assembled a team—a deep bench—of very talented, highly qualified, and richly experienced people who can address all aspects of financial planning. I'm the senior financial advisor, but we have people who specialize in tax planning, incorporation, financing, wills and powers of attorney, estate planning, insurance issues, pension planning, wealth management—for any aspect of finance, we can bring in an expert to work on your behalf. And we regularly consult with dentist clients who keep us well apprised of the issues that crop up in their practices. We're not dentists at the Leighton team, but we want to be able to speak the same language and continue to be informed."

"I'm really pleased to hear that!" said Dr. Malhotra. "In conversations with my friends and family who aren't dentists, I often feel like it's grade-school career day when people find out I'm a dentist. They have no real idea what my working day is like. So, I'm relieved to hear you know a great deal more about dentists than most others do."

Paul had worked with dozens of dentists, young and old, and he knew many walked through his door looking for a silver bullet—a one-time fix for their practices. Many, especially young dentists like Dr. Malhotra, had expected that they could go forward doing it all by themselves, informed only by their sessions with Paul. It was as if someone who visited a dentist for a filling presumed to be able to treat his own cavities. Paul sensed that Dr. Malhotra would easily understand that this wasn't a reasonable approach, and he didn't dwell on it. Rather, he emphasized the convenience and efficiencies that the Leighton team offered.

"It sounds like you spend a lot of time running around," Paul said.

A road-weary Dr. Malhotra nodded his silent agreement. "I do. It's getting tiring to say the least. And it'd be nice to have time to do other things, to be perfectly honest."

> *If you were to try to put together your own team—your own accountant, your own lawyer, your own insurance expert—there would be a lot more running around, and it would require a lot of time and effort to coordinate.*

"If you were to try to put together your own team—your own accountant, your own lawyer, your own insurance expert—there would be a lot more running around, and it would require a lot of time and effort to coordinate. Tackling the business of your work in this way would be difficult to do and much harder to do well. Our approach is comprehensive. At the very least, our full-service consulting is time-efficient; it's the most effective way to look after your finances. When everyone is working from the same file, nothing falls through the cracks, nothing is overlooked, and every possible strategy is considered."

Dr. Malhotra considered this for a moment. "I can see what you mean. I hardly have time to get to and from work, let alone fit in time to see four or five different people in as many different places. This is an interesting idea you guys have here—kind of like one-stop shopping. That concept works for me."

"I thought it might," said Paul, smiling. "We believe we'll know your situation and needs better than five people, six people, or even more who are working independently. And, in a similar fashion—just as we know you better—we know your field much better. What are the chances that any accountant or any lawyer with his shingle out has worked exclusively with dentists for an extended period? At the Leighton team, there's no learning curve because we've made dentists our business. Our business is to understand your needs and then work toward achieving them."

All this sounded reassuring to Dr. Malhotra. Though he'd have been loath to admit it, sometimes he felt overwhelmed, if not over his head, when shuffling his paperwork. When he dropped off his files with the local tax preparer in April, he was simply relieved to put it behind him. He didn't even consider the possibility that the tax preparer might have missed an opportunity for him. Dr. Malhotra went to him mostly for arithmetic, not financial advice, and that was all he could reasonably expect. Could Dr. Malhotra have missed something in prepping his files? At that point, he'd have bet on it.

"Okay," Paul said reaching into his desk drawer, "I want you to take a few minutes to do an exercise that I ask all our clients to do when we're meeting for the first time."

Dr. Malhotra must have cast a skeptical look that he wasn't aware of.

"Don't worry," Paul said as he slid a pad of paper and a pen across his desk. "This won't hurt a bit."

Chuckling, Dr. Malhotra took the pen in his hand and waited for the instructions.

"I want you to write down what concerns you most about your finances. There's a lot we can do for you in the long run, but right now, what is it you'd like to walk away with when you leave here today? What would you like us to do for you? If it's a few things, try to put the most important one first and then list the rest in descending order."

Dr. Malhotra smiled as he bent over the page. The first line was going to be easy. He took a couple of minutes to draw up the list.

Five minutes later, Paul said, "Time's up."

Dr. Malhotra set his pen down and stood up to stretch. He walked over to a credenza that had a pitcher of water and poured himself a glass. "Seems just like yesterday," he said laughing. He walked back to the table and slid the page across to Paul. "Did I pass or fail?"

Paul took a moment to scan the page and then said, "It's a pass, for sure. Of all the dentists I've done this with, the first line has almost always been the same. Maybe they've used different words from time to time, but they have the same sentiment."

"That predictable?"

The top line on Dr. Malhotra's page read, *Keep more of my income.*

"Like magazines in waiting rooms—you know they're going to be there," Paul said. "It's something close to a universal truth. What I can tell you—what I can guarantee, actually—is that with some planning, with just a few steps to start, we can save you tens of thousands of dollars over a few years. And the ability to address the items you've listed . . ." Paul pointed them out line by line:

- *Keep more of my income*
- *Pay down student loan*
- *Buy a home*

- *Acquire a practice*
- *Provide some security for parents in their retirement*

Paul continued. "The ability to accomplish these goals arises from positioning yourself properly to keep more of the income you generate. Reaching these goals rides on the management of the additional income that we can set aside."

"

The ability to accomplish your goals arises from positioning yourself properly to keep more of the income you generate.

"

Dr. Malhotra was encouraged by what he was hearing but wanted to know more.

"Before we get to that and all the other items on your list, let's do the X-ray, as I call it," Paul said. "Let's have a look at your paperwork."

Chapter 6: His life on paper

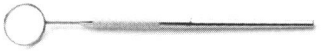

Dr. Malhotra forced a smile and pushed his file across the table. Paul flipped through the documents and made more notes. The asset side of the page was easy to look after: Dr. Malhotra had $47,800 in Registered Retirement Savings Plan (RRSPs), and a high-mileage Golf worth $8,000, less than half of what he'd originally paid for it. It wasn't complicated. He didn't own a home. Paul asked him why.

"I decided to put off that type of commitment until I felt my career was well-established and I had socked away a decent down payment. The yo-yoing of home prices scares me, and I want to wait until the market settles—the worst thing is playing the market, and then having the market play you. This happened to a friend of mine."

Dr. Malhotra was even more averse to risk when it came to putting money in the stock market. He'd read the business pages, but, as with most things, he wasn't inclined to think of himself as an expert. He made distinctions: He was a professional dentist and an amateur chef. On investing, he didn't consider himself an amateur so much as an innocent. He'd heard stories from the dentist with whom he shared the office in Strathroy—stories of dentists and other professionals who paid for their aggressive investing with almost the sum of their considerable life savings.

"Okay, but home buying adds to your net worth, so we need to get rid of our fears and accept the realities of the market. We're here to help guide you, so you're not alone. I see you've managed to lock away an impressive sum in RRSPs in a short period of time." Paul made immediate note of that. "You'll want to keep contributing like you have so far," Paul told him. "I'm sure you're aware of the tax savings you get in the short run, but the long run implications are significant too. You could potentially withdraw funds from the RRSP at a lower tax rate than when you deposited them, and that would be another tax savings. And if you were looking at buying a home, you could withdraw $25,000 for a down payment under the Home Buyers' Plan."

"

Home buying adds to your net worth.

"

"That strategy seems like a common sense approach," Dr. Malhotra said.

The RRSPs represented the vast majority of his assets. As an associate, he didn't have a sum to assign to the value of a dental practice—he was still working through the early phase of his career. He didn't own a vacation property or a piece of commercial real estate—again, these were goals for later in his career, and he believed they were realistic but had no idea how long he'd have to wait to realize them. Before any of that, though, Dr. Malhotra had one debt to clear from the ledger: the $45,000 outstanding on student loans. The math was basic, and the numbers left Dr. Malhotra feeling nervous: his net worth was $10,800.

He was better off than many in his class at dental school. After talking to former classmates at a recent alumni event at Western, he was aware that many had graduated from dental school in great debt. According to a study he'd read a couple of years before in the Journal of the Canadian Dental Association (*JCDA*), the average Canadian dental student incurs from $24,000 to $26,000 in student debt per year of study. Many of his friends were in that range. Fortunately, he wasn't because he'd lived at home while in school and worked a summer job at his father's factory in his undergrad years. On top of that, in the first couple of years as an associate, he'd managed to significantly knock down the student loan. The friends Dr. Malhotra had met up with at that alumni event and at the dental association's spring conference were well behind him on that count. He may not have owned a home, but he felt good realizing his assets exceeded his debts.

Chapter 7: Incorporation

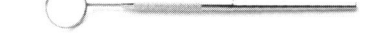

The items further down the spreadsheet were more encouraging, however. His gross income for the year was $175,000 and declared expenses were $15,000, which left him a before-tax income of $160,000.

Paul drew a deep breath. What was coming was a facts-of-life speech, one he'd given dozens of times over the course of more than a decade of working with dentists. "We should address a number of issues, but the first and foremost is the matter of incorporation," Paul said. "It's in your immediate and long-term interest to incorporate."

"How does it help?" Dr. Malhotra asked, completely thrown by the mention of incorporation. He didn't even own a practice yet, let alone was he ready to think about incorporating his practice.

"Let's start with the hard numbers, the basic personal tax rate," Paul said. "You're at the top marginal tax rate in Ontario, 46.4

percent. Almost one-quarter of your income falls into that top marginal tax rate. But the corporate rate is 15.5 percent on the first $500,000 of profit."

There was nothing subtle or ambiguous about the numbers. Paul had seen them register with almost all his clients over the years.

"That's a huge difference between the personal and corporate rates," Dr. Malhotra said.

"Especially as your profit grows over the years," Paul said. "The fact is, incorporation reduces your tax bill in the very first year, even as an associate. It becomes all the more meaningful once you own a practice and have the potential to achieve annual profits of a half-million dollars in a few years."

"

Incorporation reduces your tax bill in the very first year, even as an associate. It becomes all the more meaningful once you own a practice and have the potential to achieve annual profits of a half-million dollars in a few years.

"

"Now, the top marginal rate on dividends is 32.6 percent, and on capital gains, it's 23.2 percent. Let's set aside the capital gains for the moment. In your case, that'd apply only to the future sale of your practice, and that's something we'd like to help you with years down the line. But let's focus on the more immediate future."

Paul moved on to the issue of dividends. He'd learned over the years that, although dentistry brought all his clients together, their individual situations and circumstances varied greatly. One of the keys was identifying how to maximize the benefits of incorporation. He knew that the ability to pay out dividends, not only to the dentist but also to direct family members, would benefit Dr. Malhotra—both in the short run and the long one.

"Through incorporation, you can name direct family members as non-voting shareholders," Paul told Dr. Malhotra. "In your case, you can name your parents, but unfortunately siblings don't qualify. When you get married and have children, your spouse and your children would also be eligible to become non-voting shareholders. You'll have the ability to pay out dividends to them. The biggest advantage comes from being able to pay dividends to family members who are in a lower tax bracket than you. We'll have to take a closer look at the numbers, but you'll have significantly more money left after tax than if you'd remained unincorporated and paying tax at the top marginal rate."

The picture was becoming clearer to Dr. Malhotra. "Will you need to know about my parents' financial situation?" he asked.

"The basics should suffice. From the way you've described it, your mother has no income, so you could pay her dividends up to $40,000 per year without income tax. This could also reduce your taxes by thousands each year." Paul paused for a moment to allow the impact of this statement to sink in.

"I can't believe how much tax I could be saving. I see now how Dr. St. Louis has achieved her financial success. It must have been through prudent tax planning."

Paul nodded. "Tax planning is so much more than end-of-year numbers. With your father still working, it'd be a different story, but it might provide him a cushion in the case of early retirement."

Dr. Malhotra considered the impact of sharing dividend income with his parents. "Could there be any downside to splitting income with them?"

"We'd need to do some tax planning each year to ensure we don't compromise their tax situation. For example, parents over sixty-five who receive Old Age Security could have some or all of their government benefits clawed back if their annual income is too high. We need to be mindful of these things before deciding how much dividend income to allocate each year."

Dr. Malhotra appreciated that there were many moving parts that had to be put into place and watched closely. Nonetheless, he was encouraged by the potential long-term savings of paying dividends to family members. He envisioned a time when he might have a wife and children.

"So if and when I have children, I could start putting money aside in a trust fund for them with the dividends?" Dr. Malhotra asked.

"Well, no," Paul said. "Because of the rules in the Income Tax Act, it's not effective to allocate dividends to minor children. It only works for adult children."

The ability to save tax through dividends to family members was good, but Dr. Malhotra was disappointed that dividends couldn't be paid to minor children. Paul picked up on this. "You just need to be patient. Similar to your mother's scenario, you could pay dividends to your adult child if the child has no other income. That should be more than enough to cover their education costs each year."

Dr. Malhotra grinned and said, "Unless they want to attend dental school and follow in their father's footsteps." Paul chuckled and nodded in acknowledgement.

"What are the costs of incorporating?" Dr. Malhotra asked. He needed to know what exactly was involved before getting overly excited by the prospect.

"The costs can vary, but it's reasonable to expect fees in the $5,000 to $10,000 range to ensure it gets done properly. It's lower if you're an associate, like your situation; higher if you owned a full-fledged practice with equipment, staff, and a lease on the premises. But it's a one-time investment; it can more than pay for itself in the first year. You'll have after-tax savings far larger than that. Think of it as a financial inoculation."

"

Incorporation is a one-time investment; it can more than pay for itself in the first year.

"

Once the benefits of incorporation were covered, Paul laid out Dr. Malhotra's wish list on the table in front of him again:

- *Keep more of my income*
- *Pay down student loan*
- *Buy a home*
- *Acquire a practice*
- *Provide some security for parents in their retirement*

"I'm confident that you'll have a successful practice that will enable you to achieve all of the goals you outlined," Paul said, tapping his pen against the paper Dr. Malhotra had written on. "Just by coming here and the care you've taken with this, it's clear you have an attention to detail that will serve you well in your career and life."

Dr. Malhotra smiled and appreciated the compliment.

"And I'm equally confident that the savings you'll accrue with effective tax planning will put you in a position to pay off your student debt promptly. You're in a good position, you really are. We can look after this loan soon."

Paul pointed to the third item on his list: *Buy a home.* "Some dentists in your age group who work with us don't own homes," Paul said. "Others are looking to pay down the mortgages on their first homes as quickly as possible. Through incorporation, you can benefit and speed up the process of saving for a down payment or paying off the mortgage sooner. The prudent mix of salary and dividends will leave much more money than you would have had available if you weren't incorporated."

"

The prudent mix of salary and dividends will leave much more money than you would have had available if you weren't incorporated.

"

"What are the other implications if I incorporate?" Dr. Malhotra asked.

"It's important to register the Professional Corporation with the dental college and renew the registration annually. Incorporation limits your liability to creditors but not your professional liability. More importantly, additional after-tax income would be available to pay a corporate debt, a scenario that would play out with the purchase of a practice. In my experience, incorporated dentists can pay off such debts in about two-thirds the time that unincorporated ones require. This could save thousands of dollars of interest and improve cash flow in the practice years earlier."

"I've often worried about how I'll manage the debt load of a home and a practice early in my career. I guess incorporation will provide me with opportunities to help achieve my goals sooner than I thought possible. But what other areas of my financial plan should I address right away?"

> *Incorporated dentists can pay off debts in about two-thirds the time that unincorporated ones require. This could save thousands of dollars of interest and improve cash flow in the practice years earlier.*

"Well, in the short term, we should look at drawing up a will and powers of attorney. We'll introduce you to an estate planning lawyer to draft the estate documents. Then we'll do a thorough insurance analysis to ensure you have adequate coverage in place. In the long term, you'll want to look at establishing a dental practice or perhaps purchasing one. When we get there, I'd review the price of the future practice and compare it to the cash flow the practice could generate. This will allow us to get a handle on how long it would take to repay the debt to purchase a practice or set up a new one. Down the road, it may even include buying a commercial property for your practice."

Dr. Malhotra had a lot to take in, and though he tried not to let on, he was a bit overwhelmed. He realized that, even though he'd been scrupulous and thorough in his handling of the day-to-day aspects of his finances, he hadn't spent enough time looking ahead. He'd always presumed that if he handled the day-to-day, the future would look after itself.

As their session wound down, Paul made sure that Dr. Malhotra understood that the tax planning team was just that—a team made up of specialists in financing, insurance issues, and legal matters.

"It's not that you'd be handed off to one tax planner," Paul said. "We're the sum of our parts. We all work within our individual expertise, and though we may not be dentists, we do our best to understand you."

Paul sat back and tried to recount how many times he'd sat across from a dentist who was making his first trip into the Leighton team's office. Paul was confident he could put Dr. Malhotra on a track that would more rapidly build his net worth and protect his financial interests, and those of his family.

"You've made a wise move taking this step to manage your finances before they manage you. From what I can see here," Paul said, tapping on the file folder in front of him, "and by what you've told me, I know we can come up with a few strategies."

"I really think you can, too. I'm glad I made the call and came to see you today. I almost thought of cancelling, I was so hesitant to discuss these things."

Paul gave Dr. Malhotra some reading to take home with him and suggested they set up a meeting for the following week. "Sleep on it, and if you give me the green light, we can get the ball rolling," he said.

Chapter 8: New beginnings

Dr. Malhotra went over to his parents' home for dinner that night. He didn't tell them about the meeting or, at least, nothing more than saying that he'd met with an accountant. His father seemed impressed. He did, however, send an e-mail message to Dr. St. Louis when he made it back to his apartment that night.

Adeline, hello.

I met with Paul Leighton today. It went well, I think, but it's an awful lot to take in. I don't know if my head was quite spinning when I came out of there, but as he laid it out for me, the possibilities and approaches sounded promising. I think that there are benefits there for my finances—as Paul said, some in the long run, but some others pretty quickly. I want to thank you for passing along the information about the Leighton team.

Arjun

Later that night, Dr. St. Louis sent a short note back.

> *Arjun, it was my pleasure if I was able to be of any help. I'm sure that you were more fully in command of the discussion of business and personal finance than I was. I had my husband along, but he's a professor in the classics department, not the business school. He had an even harder time keeping up than I did, and neither of us had ever done a business class in school, not even in high school. That said, I've tried to take a more informed interest ever since. I'm no expert—I know enough to trust the experts—but I look at things differently now. As for seeing benefits for your finances, I've come around to thinking that, to a great degree, they're integrated . . . that is, if they're not one and the same.*

Dr. Malhotra read the last line twice and thought about it. He typed a reminder into the day planner in his BlackBerry: *Call Leighton team, schedule meeting.*

At lunch the next day, Dr. Malhotra did just that. Paul was pleased to hear he'd made the decision to move forward, and they arranged to meet early the following week. He was told to bring along his financial information again so that the team could have a copy on file. Paul also gave him a piece of homework to finish before he arrived: a precise workup on his month-to-month expenses and spending habits.

"We really need to see what you can live comfortably on, so be honest," Paul told him. "I know many people are inclined to understate these things . . . maybe they just don't want to seem spendthrift or extravagant. But in drawing up a budget, we need an honest idea of what you need to live on. The objective isn't to curb your lifestyle spending, but to work with it for our planning assumptions."

Dr. Malhotra knew he'd have to review his expenses to get a better understanding of how he spent his money each month—not just the typical expenses, but the discretionary ones as well, such as cooking gadgets and coffees ordered out.

"Sure thing. I can do that. I'm looking forward to our meeting."

As soon as he got home that evening, Dr. Malhotra logged into his bank account online, printed the past year's account history, and started organizing his expenses. He'd do the same with his credit card bills. As he was going to be a while, he plugged in the kettle, turned on the radio, and settled in for a couple of hours of work.

Dr. Malhotra returned to the Leighton offices a week later. He felt more self-assured about this trip. In the days leading up to the first meeting, he'd puzzled over the acronyms for the various investments and saving plans. His homework this time didn't test his knowledge of matters he'd only glanced at in brochures bulk mailed from banks.

He'd literally done his homework. He'd studied the website set up by the Leighton team and pored over the case studies that were available there. Many of them focused on financial planning for dentists who were well-established in their practices, dentists like Dr. St. Louis, but it gave him much to think about. There were also case studies concerning issues that could be important much later on in his career but were simply matters of curiosity right now—for example, the implications of an associate joining a practice, or the potential to finance the purchase of a second practice using corporate savings and without bank financing.

There were also several case studies about dentists in circumstances similar to his own, and Dr. Malhotra had become more aware of the benefits of shrewd financial planning and felt more confident in his ability to discuss the issues with Paul. In reading some of the case studies involving more experienced dentists who hadn't incorporated and effectively planned their finances, Dr. Malhotra had realized that he was starting off on the right foot.

The written portion of the assignment Paul had given him in advance of their second meeting was a task he'd taken seriously: *Get a good read of what you can live comfortably on.* He'd prepped the assignment as meticulously as he had assignments in school. He'd gone to his chequebook to get a precise dollar value on his insurance and calculated his gas expenses based on the mileage he'd put on the Golf over the past year, since he'd last had the car in for a tune-up. He'd factored in two oil changes that he should have had over that time and put in an estimate for repairs. He hadn't yet had to worry about repairs—he'd been lucky dodging that bullet—but he knew his luck couldn't possibly keep up.

He'd looked at past banking statements to get an idea of what he spent at the supermarket on his twice-weekly trips. He'd also looked at those statements to see how often he dined out—more often than he'd thought. He'd combed his memory to think of gifts he'd bought family and friends. At the bottom of the page, he'd made note of the cost of leasing a car that would make his commute to Strathroy and Kitchener more comfortable and, in winter, likely safer. He was happy in his apartment and planned on staying until he purchased his own home. He didn't have anything fancy, just some hand-me-down pieces from his parents' place.

Paul came out and greeted him. "So, did you really sink your teeth into the assignment I gave you?"

"I did. I learned quite a bit," Dr. Malhotra said as he handed Paul the folder with the information.

"Very comprehensive," Paul said. "Many clients—maybe even most—who fill out these forms round figures off and usually round them off on the low side. And with the idea of sheltering as much income as possible from taxes, many clients provide estimates of living expenses that are just too low. It's counterproductive to submit a budget that you just live on. It defeats what we're trying to do. The budget has to be realistic. We're not looking for *sacrifice* . . . we're simply looking for *control* or, more precisely, *self-control.*"

Dr. Malhotra was comfortable with this idea and, maybe more importantly, well-practiced at it. He wasn't so far removed from his days when he'd lived on a shoestring as a student in dental school. While others would go out for lunch, he'd have brought something from home. When others were going out at night, he'd be at home cooking. His former classmates occasionally ribbed Dr. Malhotra about his conservative streak. They called him a "low-flier."

Dr. Malhotra had taken to heart Paul's words from their first meeting. He'd left some breathing room. He'd budgeted for a vacation—a vacation that he wanted to take this year. He wasn't about to spend a couple of weeks close to home again. He'd also budgeted for a few pieces of new furniture and some kitchenware he'd spotted on his last trip to the Williams-Sonoma store in Toronto. Paul Leighton wasn't used to seeing $2,500 allotted for cookware. But then again, he knew that it was better that the young dentist include these items on his budget rather than purchase the items on some sort of impulse outside the pocket money that the budget accounted for.

"So you think you could live comfortably on an after-tax income of $60,000?"

"I do. It should give me what I need to be comfortable. Nothing excessive, but not wanting for much either."

Paul did some quick math, then laid out the rough numbers as he'd promised at the last meeting. Dr. Malhotra didn't have to look very hard at the two columns to find a significant difference. He could tell by the number that Paul circled at the bottom of the page that his financial picture for the year ahead would look vastly different than the past calendar year.

The difference in his total taxes paid between his unincorporated practice and his practice after incorporation was $22,800 per year.

"That's your tax deferral," said Paul, "And it shows how much your cash flow can improve immediately. These are the very basics. We haven't started to talk about the benefits of RRSPs, or the ability to pay out dividends to non-voting shareholders. We're only starting to scratch the surface here.

"These types of savings become much greater as your practice becomes more established and the gross income grows. It's reasonable to look at this as a starting point, and to believe that when we go through your records and crunch your numbers, we might find savings elsewhere—one place to start would be your expenses."

> *When you're in a position to buy a home, you'll be able to withdraw a tax-free amount from an RRSP under the Home Buyer's Plan to put toward a down payment.*

"One thing that I have thought about before is if part of my travel can be deducted," said Dr. Malhotra. "I do a lot of travelling to get from one practice to the other. I'd also like to know if I can get a write-down on my car expenses."

SECTION I: DR. MALHOTRA'S EDUCATION

"Yes, we'll look at that," Paul answered. "These are good points. I'm impressed! Being able to deduct all eligible expenses is to your advantage and again a tax savings—something to explore." Paul moved on to the longer term implications after incorporation.

"We'd have you contribute to an RRSP. You'd see an immediate tax savings and tax-deferred growth for years to come. And, when you're in a position to buy a home, you'll be able to withdraw a tax-free amount from your RRSP under the Home Buyer's Plan to put toward a down payment."

"

Over the lifetime of dental equipment, the tax advantages between ownership and leasing are the same; however, the cost of financing is usually less than the cost of leasing.

"

Paul and Dr. Malhotra looked at issues that might come up over the course of a couple of years. One day he'd look at setting up a practice, and Paul recommended he buy equipment rather than lease it. Paul explained that over the lifetime of the equipment, the tax advantages between ownership and leasing would be the same; however, the cost of financing was usually less than the cost of leasing. There also would be less control over the leased equipment. Paul could recount many incidents when dentists had leased costly equipment, such as lasers or CAD/CAM machines, only to find they couldn't resell them until the end of the lease if they were underutilized and collecting dust.

They also discussed matters that were sure to come up further down the line, such as purchasing a home or purchasing a commercial building for the practice. They even discussed financial strategies for the far-off future, such as how incorporation could serve not just his parents' interests but also those of a family of his own.

"Whoa, you've gone far off into the future! But I see what you're getting at," said Dr. Malhotra, laughing, but delighted to be considering such things.

"It's exciting to focus on long-term objectives; however, we need to manage your risk," Paul replied. "It's imperative that you protect your ability to earn an income, so we need to spend some time talking about disability and critical illness policies. We also need to plan your estate. A will and powers of attorney are necessary and so is life insurance to cover your debt."

"

Life policies should be owned and paid by your company; it's a more efficient use of cash flow. Because the corporate tax rate is less than the top personal tax rate, there's more money left over to pay the insurance premium.

"

Paul laid the numbers out on paper for adequate coverage.

"Life policies should be owned and paid by your company; it's a more efficient use of cash flow. Because the corporate tax rate is less than the top personal tax rate, there's more money left over to pay the insurance premium." He then further discussed what would be the standard application and underwriting process.

Over the course of the hour, Dr. Malhotra began to envision how his life could change. He couldn't resist looking to the future, to the potential benefits that he could reap from long-term financial planning. He felt that things were really coming together and all the parts of the puzzle were finally meshing. He didn't have so much to feel insecure about anymore.

In the end, Dr. Malhotra informed Paul he wished to retain the services of the Leighton team. Paul was pleased and explained the options available. Dr. Malhotra chose to start with the Tax Saver Plan. This meant they would continue with further analysis of what they'd already started: income tax and incorporation, as well as a comprehensive personal financial plan, insurance and estate planning, and debt and financial arrangements. Dr. Malhotra believed (and Paul concurred) that it would be time to rework the plan in a couple of years when Dr. Malhotra was looking to finance a home, start a family, purchase a practice, or execute some sort of significant career move that would require additional expert support.

"I'll put you in touch with a lawyer who specializes in setting up Professional Corporations for dentists. It'll ensure you benefit from the tax savings we discussed as soon as possible. I'll also arrange meetings with our estate lawyer for the will and powers of attorney, and with our insurance advisor to get your coverage in place," Paul said.

Shaking hands with Paul, Dr. Malhotra replied, "Yes, this is all terrific. My parents will finally be able to make trips home to visit my aunts and uncles and cousins." He saw it as a way to repay them for all the help they had given him. The financial help he was about to get from Paul and the other members of the Leighton team would ensure that his kids wouldn't be eating macaroni and cheese or ramen noodles in their college residences.

A couple of weeks later, Dr. Malhotra received an e-mail from the Leighton team's corporate law specialist confirming that Dr. Arjun Malhotra Dentistry Professional Corporation was now registered with the dental college. Going forward, he'd be drawing a salary from the corporate cash flow.

Dr. Malhotra's life didn't change very much over the next few months. He did have to inform the dental offices where he worked to direct his income to the new Professional Corporation instead of to him personally, but otherwise his lifestyle saw no significant changes. Even though he knew there were financial benefits available to him, he remained cautious.

He tracked his expenses more closely and resisted most, if not all, material temptation (though he did finally purchase the stand mixer he'd always wanted). The most profound change in his life, though, was Anita Sharma, a hygienist who worked in the Kitchener dental office where he was an associate. They'd chatted occasionally and eaten together at the staff summer barbecue the previous year, but it wasn't until he saw on paper what his future could look like that he finally realized he could move ahead with the bigger things in life, such as dating, marriage, and kids. He asked her out for coffee one week and lunch at a bistro close to work the next week. By the third week, he'd managed enough courage to invite her to his apartment, where he cooked her a spicy Indian curry that impressed her so much she pleaded with him to make it for her mother the following weekend.

Dr. Malhotra had moved forward in many ways.

Chapter 9: Tweaking the plan

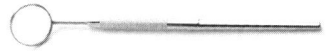

Dr. Malhotra had worked with the Leighton team for a little less than a year and was already starting to see returns on his bottom line. He was pleased with his progress towards paying off the student debt, and that he was able to support his parents by paying them dividends. Dr. Malhotra felt less stressed about his career and his life away from the office. He'd never put it down on paper or even talked about it with family or friends, although he'd discussed it with Anita a little bit, but he did have something like a five-year plan for buying a home and practice and settling down. Dr. Malhotra felt like he was taking control of his finances, but a couple of events happened that he couldn't have foreseen.

First, Dr. Tarber, the principal dentist at the London practice where Dr. Malhotra was an associate, got ill. An alumnus of the University of Western Ontario, Dr. Tarber had given many recent graduates an opportunity to work as associates at his practice over the years. One day at the office, not long after his fiftieth birthday, he'd felt a tremor in his hand. He'd thought nothing of it—perhaps he'd pinched a nerve sailing—but it persisted. After seeing his family doctor and undergoing tests, he was diagnosed with early-onset Parkinson's. Dr. Tarber needed Dr. Malhotra to cover for him fulltime to look after his long-standing patients, and Dr. Malhotra was pleased and agreed quite readily. Because he couldn't work anywhere else while he filled in for Dr. Tarber, a couple of recent graduates filled in for him on days he was to work in Kitchener and Strathroy.

Early on in Dr. Tarber's treatment, his condition stabilized, but it didn't improve. It was clear he wouldn't be physically able to continue with his practice. He stated his intention to put it up for sale, and because of their relationship, Dr. Tarber would give Dr. Malhotra the first chance at buying it. It was an ideal opportunity for Dr. Malhotra in every way—except timing. He felt it was simply too soon.

Things were also happening quickly for Dr. Malhotra away from the office. His relationship with Anita was growing more serious. Dr. Malhotra liked that she understood the pressures of his work and shared his love of food—she was even more accomplished than he was in the kitchen. Within the first year of dating, they were engaged and Anita was giving her fiancé a not-so-subtle push for them to buy a home rather than move into his somewhat cramped apartment or look for another apartment to rent.

"We can't possibly get all of my stuff in your little apartment, and what's the point in moving to another apartment when we're likely to move again after we get married? We should buy now and move once," Anita reasoned.

So it was no wonder that Dr. Malhotra had real concerns when he went to see Paul. News of Dr. Tarber's desire to sell his practice and the pressure he was feeling from Anita to buy a home in London was more than he could handle. He needed some advice, and from a professional who could look past the emotional aspects of both situations.

"Paul, good to see you again. I have a lot to discuss with you!"

"That's what we're here for. So, tell me what's going on with you, Arjun."

"Anita, my fiancée—"

"Congratulations! That's wonderful news," said Paul, truly pleased to hear of the progress happening in Dr. Malhotra's life.

"Thank you. Anita wants to buy a house, now. I didn't even feel comfortable about taking out a student loan, but the idea of carrying huge debts on a practice *and* a property—well, I'm going to go grey in a hurry!" Dr. Malhotra chuckled. "I don't know how it's doable. As for the opportunity I told you about on the phone, I need to see if I can manage the price that Dr. Tarber is talking about, around $750,000. And in terms of house prices, we've only started to look casually, but once we see something, I want to know what I can afford. We're lucky because Anita and I have savings that we could use toward a down payment, but still, it's hard to see trying to manage a practice or a house, never mind both."

"I've seen lots of dentists get into trouble with big debts," Paul said. "Inevitably, though, the real problems came when they didn't have a strategy for managing their cash flow. There are ways to do it and ways not to—rules of thumb that you should try to follow and traps that you have to avoid."

"Okay," said Dr. Malhotra rather skeptically.

"Let me show you some numbers on paper so you can actually see how this might work." First, Paul wrote down *100%* on a blank page. "These days, banks are prepared to provide 100 percent financing on the purchase of a practice. They're more than happy to do that because dental practices are a safe bet. They're even willing to extend loans over a ten-year period, with interest-only payments through the first year or two. Doing that alone would allow you to defer in the neighbourhood of $75,000 in the first year."

"Payments of $75,000 per year?" asked Dr. Malhotra. "That sounds like a lot. How could I afford that?"

"It should be quite affordable. Practice values reflect the cash flow generated by the business," Paul explained. "Did you bring a copy of Dr. Tarber's financial statements with you today?"

"

Banks are prepared to provide 100 percent financing on the purchase of a dental practice. They're even willing to extend loans over a ten-year period, with interest-only payments through the first year or two.

"

Dr. Malhotra handed Paul a folder of information related to the practice purchase that he had been maintaining. After reviewing the financial statements for a moment, Paul wrote down some numbers on the page again. Paul showed Dr. Malhotra how he could take out a loan and still maintain his current income. There would be enough cash flow to make the required loan payments, cover his corporate taxes *and* pay off his practice loan faster. In due time, he could issue dividends to pay off a future house mortgage.

As Dr. Malhotra reviewed the numbers on the page, he began to see the practice as something he might be able to afford. "I'm not sure I'd be able to navigate my way through the books, the loan applications, and negotiations. And where would I find the time?"

"Don't jump the gun yet. Hear me out. The only way we can say for sure if Dr. Tarber's asking price is reasonable is to have a professional valuation completed. A valuator will look over the practice's books, equipment, and patient charts to determine a fair value. We can suggest a couple of firms who specialize in valuing dental practices," Paul said. "If we think it's a good opportunity and a good price for you, then we could pursue financing."

"Two big-ticket items at a time, though—that's the problem I'm having trouble finding resolution to," Dr. Malhotra said.

"Well, it's how you balance them," Paul said. "We know from past experience that the cash flow from the practice is more than enough to cover the payments on the loan. It helps that the interest is tax-deductible.

> "
>
> *Focus on paying non-deductible debt before tax-deductible debt.*
>
> "

"With a new home, we first recommend you put 20 percent down, with full prepayment privileges. What we're really aiming for in a situation like this is to pay down the non-deductible interest before the deductible interest. We'd have you pay down your house more quickly than you're paying off your practice. The extra cash flow we talked about—the $75,000—could be redirected to your mortgage instead of the practice loan. This amount could be quite high while interest-only payments continue on the practice loan.

"Each year, of course, we have to review your debts to determine how we can continue to stretch out the practice payments and use the extra cash flow to pay off the mortgage first. In other words, focus on paying non-deductible debt before tax-deductible debt.

Almost inevitably, when a dentist gets into financial trouble, it's because cash flow hasn't been managed well or the non-deductible and tax-deductible debts haven't been addressed properly."

Dr. Malhotra and Paul played around with the numbers for another fifteen minutes. They were able to set a target for the home purchase and establish that he'd be able to make an offer pending a valuation of Dr. Tarber's practice.

> *Almost inevitably, when a dentist gets into financial trouble, it's because the cash flow hasn't been managed well or the non-deductible and tax-deductible debts haven't been addressed properly.*

"I know it's a lot on your plate, and it'll be tough at the beginning, but with a game plan and the resolve to stick to it, you'll achieve all these things and more."

"You're right, and I see that now. Thanks again for setting me on the right course, Paul. Maybe I can do both, after all."

Dr. Arjun Malhotra, DDS

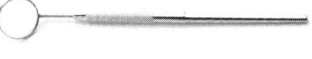

The Associate

- 30 years old

- Graduated 2 years ago from Schulich School of Medicine & Dentistry at University of Western Ontario

- Been associating since graduation in three locations: London, Kitchener, and Strathroy

- Engaged to be married to Anita Sharma, a hygienist from the Kitchener practice

- Considering the purchase of Dr. Tarber's dental practice in London

For the first time in his professional life, Dr. Malhotra had a plan for the future. The following is a summary of the numbers behind the plan.

Goals

- Reduce taxes
- Pay down student debt
- Purchase first home
- Establish a new practice
- Security for parents

Cash Flow

Gross Associate Income	$175,000
Business Expenses	($15,000)
Income Before Taxes	$160,000
Personal Tax & Canada Pension Plan (CPP)	($58,000)
Net Cash Flow (before incorporation)	**$102,000**

Net Worth

ASSETS

Vehicle	$8,000
Registered Retirement Savings Plan (RRSP)	$47,800
	$55,800

LIABILITIES

Student Loan	$45,000
	$45,000

NET WORTH	**$10,800**

Incorporation, Tax Reduction & Cash Flow Improvement

Establish a Professional Corporation, with Dr. Malhotra as the voting common shareholder, and parents as non-voting common shareholders for ability to receive dividends.

	Sole Proprietor	Incorporated
Revenue	$175,000	$175,000
Expenses	($15,000)	($15,000)
Salary to Dr. Malhotra		($81,000)
Employer CPP		($2,200)
Corporate Taxes		($12,000)
Corporate Income after tax		$64,800
Personal Income to Dr. Malhotra	$160,000	$81,000
Personal Tax & CPP*	($58,000)	($21,000)
Net Cash Flow	**$102,000**	**$124,800**
TAX REDUCTION / CASH FLOW IMPROVEMENT		**$22,800**

Cash flow is increased as total taxes are reduced by $22,800 per year.

The remaining corporate profit of $64,800 could be paid as dividends to pay off student loan, provide support to parents, or pay the mortgage.

* For simplicity, RRSP contributions have been excluded from this illustration.

Surplus Cash Flow over Two Years (prior to practice purchase)

Annual Dividends to Parents	$64,800
Tax at parents' marginal tax rate (@ 15%)	($9,800)
Annual after-tax cash flow	**$55,000**
Total after two years	**$110,000**

Use of Cash Flow (from above)

Repayment of Student Loan	$45,000
Financial Support to Parents	$15,000
Surplus Savings for Home Purchase	$50,000
	$110,000

Within two years, Dr. Malhotra paid off his student loan, began providing financial support for his parents, and built up the down payment amount necessary for a home purchase.

Home Downpayment (prior to practice purchase)

Objective is to purchase a home valued at $500,000. Downpayment should be 20% (or $100,000).

RRSP Home Buyer's Plan - Arjun Malhotra	$25,000
RRSP Home Buyer's Plan - Anita Sharma	$25,000
Surplus Savings for Home Purchase	$50,000
DOWNPAYMENT (20% of purchase price)	**$100,000**

Purchase of Dental Practice

Projections illustrate there is enough cash flow to cover the principal payments and provide a generous surplus. The surplus can be issued as dividends to Dr. Malhotra to pay down his home mortgage first, and later to repay the practice loan once the home is paid off.

Purchase Price	**$750,000**
Revenue	$800,000
Expenses (@ 55% of revenue)	($440,000)
Interest on Practice Loan	($24,000)
Salary to Dr. Malhotra*	($125,000)
Employer CPP	($2,200)
Corporate Taxes	($32,300)
Corporate Income after tax	**$176,500**
Principal Loan Payments ($750,000 over 10 years)	**$75,000**
Dividends or debt repayment	**$101,500**
	$176,500

Surplus of $176,500 can be used as dividends towards the mortgage or retained in the company to pay the pratice loan.

*salary capped at $125,000 to allow maximum RRSP contributions.

Mortgage Repayment (after practice purchase)

Assuming Dr. Malhotra can negotiate interest-only payments for the first two years of the practice loan, all surplus cash flow can be paid as dividends and directed to his mortgage. Practice loan payments of $75,000 to begin in the third year.

Balance of Mortgage	**$400,000**
Year 1 dividends ($176,500 net of tax @ 32.6%)	$119,000
Year 2 dividends ($176,500 net of tax @ 32.6%)	$119,000
Year 3 dividends ($101,500 net of tax @ 32.6%)	$68,500
Year 4 dividends ($101,500 net of tax @ 32.6%)	$68,500
Year 5 dividends ($37,000 net of tax @ 32.6%)	$25,000
	$400,000

Home fully paid off in 5 years.

Results

- Taxes reduced by $22,800 per year and cash flow improved

- $64,800 paid as dividends to parents at their low marginal tax rates for the first two years from corporate profit

- $45,000 student loan paid off in Year 1

- $500,000 mortagage and down payment paid off in five years

- Purchases $750,000 dental practice in London and has enough surplus to pay down practice loan principal and interest after five years as home mortgage is paid off first

Section II: Dr. Bekker's Struggles

Chapter 10: A step in the right direction

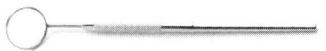

Dr. Bekker could hardly believe that it was the ODA's annual spring meeting again. It seemed like only a couple of months had passed since the last one—when the BMW broke down. There'd been a series of household crises since then. If it wasn't his son's computer needing replacement, then it was needing to call in the plumber, the roofer, or the electrician, or the twins needing help filling out their applications to university, arguing about what schools to attend (and not together). If it weren't these and any number of other things that cropped up, such as his wife reminding him on a weekly basis how they hadn't gone on vacation in a while, it was something else. There was no rest from the chaos of kids, marriage, house ownership, and running a dental practice.

One year was much like the others, and just when he felt like things were *almost* under control, something always seemed to go off the rails, more frantic than actually tragic. Most of the time it was on the home front, and so it was again in early spring when the twins were waiting for—fingers crossed—acceptance letters from the universities they had finally applied to. Of course, they couldn't pick something close to home, which would have meant substantial savings for Dr. Bekker (as in, the twins could live at home, rent-free). Vancouver and Calgary definitely weren't close to home.

This year, though, he also had some concerns about his practice. His lease was entering its final year, and he was dreading the renegotiating process that usually ensued at the end of such tenancy agreements. It simply wasn't one of his talents. He'd heard horror stories from others who'd leased space in the same building, and a couple of medical specialists had decided the easiest course of action was to relocate their practices. Dr. Bekker couldn't completely rule that option out, even if he did dread the thought of moving. In the end, he knew he'd sign, feeling like he'd been squeezed again. Owning his own space would be less hassle, but he couldn't see how it'd be possible, and he hardly had the time to give it any real thought.

Getting to this year's meeting wouldn't be as challenging as it had been last year. Riding school was rained out that morning, and the twins were getting a ride to school from a friend. For once, Dr. Bekker was early.

His wife, Trish, managed the dental office. She mostly looked after appointments, billings, and assorted paperwork. With her husband off for the day, she booked a couple of morning appointments downtown—the doctor for a checkup and a round of shopping for some après-ski wear in advance of taking the girls to the slopes for spring break. She was going to drop him off at the Metro Toronto Convention Centre, where the conference was being held again this year.

"Remember last year the BMW conked out on me? I like this a lot better, Trish. And I get front-door service!"

Trish Bekker came to a stop in front of the convention centre and leaned over to kiss her husband goodbye. "I'll see you tonight for dinner?"

"I think so. I'll call if I'm late. Don't spend too much time playing hooky," Dr. Bekker said teasingly as he shut the door. He made his way to the coffee bar for a necessary morning jolt. After he ordered a large Columbian, Dr. Bekker noticed that Dr. Malhotra was sitting down with a newspaper, a yogurt, and a coffee. Dr. Bekker walked right up beside him.

"You'll be relieved to know that you won't have to give me a boost today," Dr. Bekker said. "I didn't have to drive in myself."

Dr. Malhotra looked up and smiled when he recognized Dr. Bekker. "Dr. Bekker, good to see you again. I have my cables with me just in case."

Dr. Bekker couldn't quite remember Dr. Malhotra's name. "I'm sorry, but it's . . ." he said.

"Arjun," Dr. Malhotra finished for him.

"Things are going well for you, I hope," Dr. Bekker said. He wasn't in command of all of the details of their conversation from a year ago. "You're in Kitchener, right? But then I want to say some other place, too. Please help me out."

"I'm an associate with a practice in Kitchener, but I'm based in London," Dr. Malhotra said. "And things are going on quite nicely. No complaints."

No complaints. That was almost taunting, given Dr. Bekker's state of mind. He wouldn't have known where to start; he had so many complaints to tally off.

"In fact, I have good news to share with you," Dr. Malhotra continued. "I'm engaged to be married."

"Fantastic! Congratulations," said Dr. Bekker, patting Dr. Malhotra's shoulder to share his good cheer. "Marriage is great. I wish you and your bride all the best."

Over the next five minutes, the two rounded off the niceties: the wedding (Anita was diligently making plans), the business (steady as usual), and the front page of the paper (times harder for many). The last one hit home for Dr. Bekker. It just didn't seem to add up. He felt he was working harder than ever, like the treadmill under his feet was accelerating and he couldn't stay on. It was literally all he could do to keep up.

"I could use another vacation," he said, looking out the window at the grey waterfront.

"Another?" Dr. Malhotra said. "I feel lucky that I could take *one* this year."

"Where did you go? Someplace sunny, I hope!"

"I was in New York for nine days a couple of months back," he said. "I went to a cooking school there for a workshop. . .."

"Cooking! What a great skill to have. You'll make your fiancée really happy with that ability. I can't even cook an egg, how sad is that? I've tried, but they always come out tough and inedible. Hey, I guess that's why we have Denny's!" Dr. Bekker said, laughing.

"It's a hobby. It relaxes me and allows me to use my creative side for a change. And then I get to eat something good after it," Dr. Malhotra said. "I took a week-long course on Tuscan cooking. My nights were free, so I went out with a couple of friends from university and also went to two cricket matches. I made a week of it. For the first time in years, I really made time for myself. And I learned a few new recipes. My fiancée can't get enough of my *ravioli con ricotta*."

"That sounds fantastic! But even if I wanted to do something like that, I don't think I could get it by my family," Dr. Bekker said. "This year we're going to Whistler. My wife and I will ski, and the kids will snowboard and run up expenses. By the time we come back, I'll need another vacation, but I couldn't even afford the last one we took." Dr. Bekker sighed heavily and drained the last of his coffee. He had a thought: maybe the twins would like a cooking course like the one Dr. Malhotra took.

"What would a course like that cost?" he asked Dr. Malhotra.

"My nine days there . . . well, I'm not sure, but the course itself was about $3,000 US," he said.

"You could have gone to Italy for that much!"

"That's what I'm hoping to do next year or the year after—take a cooking course or two there. Get as close to authentic as possible."

Dr. Bekker was impressed. When he'd been Dr. Malhotra's age, he'd gone to Las Vegas for a few weekends with friends and to South Carolina for golf another weekend, but he'd never done anything quite so high-end as taking a cooking course in New York or Italy. A year ago, he hadn't come away with the impression that this would have been in Dr. Malhotra's price range.

At that moment, Dr. St. Louis walked into the lobby with another dentist who looked to be about forty years old, fit, and perfectly groomed in a dark and lightly pinstriped suit. The two walked up to the coffee bar when Dr. St. Louis spied her two breakfast partners from the previous year's conference.

"Arjun, Dr. Bekker, how are you?" she said. "We don't have any worries about a late start this time, do we?"

"Adeline, good to see you," Dr. Malhotra said.

As the conversation continued, it was evident to Dr. Bekker that the two other dentists had stayed in touch after that chance meeting a year ago. It wasn't just that they were on a first-name basis, but also that she knew about his engagement to Anita and his going to New York for the cooking course, and Dr. Malhotra seemed to know about the trip she'd taken with her husband to Paris last summer. He felt like a kid cut out of a high-school clique.

"Oh, pardon me. This is Dr. Trevor Parry," she said, introducing the dapper dentist standing next to her. "He joined my practice as an associate last fall."

The four exchanged pleasantries, and the two dentists from Ottawa took seats at the table with Drs. Malhotra and Bekker.

"I want to thank you again for giving me the tip about the Leighton team," Dr. Malhotra said.

Dr. Bekker was thoroughly puzzled by this. The name sounded vaguely familiar, but he couldn't place it. *A supplier? Something to do with work? Something else entirely?*

> "
>
> *It's always good to be looking a day ahead and years ahead, too.*
>
> "

"No need to thank me, Arjun," Dr. St. Louis said. "I hope everything is working out well for you."

"It's making a big difference for me already, and I know it'll pay off in the long run," Dr. Malhotra said.

"That's great," she said. She was about to say something more about her own long-term planning—how Dr. Parry was coming into her practice with the plan of buying it upon her retirement. But the timing of her retirement and the terms of the sale weren't carved in stone yet and Dr. Parry had only just been introduced to the two other dentists at the table, so she held back that bit of news. She opted for advice that could have been cribbed from a fortune cookie but that really reflected her approach to finances. "It's always good to be looking a day ahead and years ahead, too."

Dr. Bekker couldn't hold back. He had to ask Dr. Malhotra: "What was that group you mentioned?"

"The Leighton team," Dr. Malhotra said. "I asked Adeline about the people who look after her finances, and she gave me the contact information. I went to see them not long after last year's conference, and I can tell you that my financial picture looks a lot clearer and a lot brighter now. That's how I made it to New York, and it's how I'm going to get to Italy."

Dr. Bekker was curious and impressed. His approach had always been to shuffle the paperwork onto his wife's desk. She managed the office, and he didn't make any distinction between managing the office and managing their finances. He'd always assumed that if the office was handled well, the finances would look after themselves. As long as there were patients making appointments, the cash flow would be there and he and his wife would be able to make it work—it was how he'd operated for twenty years. He usually tuned out talk when it turned to finance. He golfed with friends he had known from dental school, and it seemed like the subject of their practices' finances and management always came up when he was lining up a putt, distracting him when he was trying to focus. Talk about investments and portfolios and brokers and escrow threw him off, whether it was on the golf course, at a party, or out for dinner with friends. He couldn't change the subject fast enough.

This time, though, Dr. Bekker tuned in. In part, it was because of the image he had of Dr. St. Louis and her practice. She seemed to live a comfortable life, and not only compared to his. In all truth, Dr. Bekker and his wife were always in a mad scramble to get some kind of paperwork done: billings, insurance, payroll, subscriptions, equipment. The list went on and on. He'd had enough of the chaos and realized it couldn't hurt to at least contact the outfit Dr. Malhotra had talked to. Maybe his wife could look into it and see if it was worthwhile.

"Well, it was lovely catching up, gentlemen, but we want to get an early start on the conference, so if you'll excuse us," said Dr. St. Louis, as she and Dr. Parry made their way to the main hall.

Before Dr. Malhotra decided to break away, too, Dr. Bekker seized the opportunity. "Do you know how I can get in touch with. . ." He struggled with the name.

"The Leighton team?" Dr. Malhotra said, finishing the sentence. "Here's my card. E-mail or call me, and I'll get the information for you."

He took Dr. Malhotra's business card and put it into his wallet. It stayed there for a week. By the time Dr. Bekker pulled it out and called, his outlook and circumstances had changed dramatically.

Chapter 11: Eyes wide open

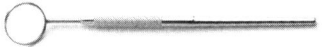

Following the ODA conference, the Bekkers flew out to Whistler for their skiing trip. Dr. Bekker's wife was an avid and expert skier and had competed at the provincial level as a teenager. Dr. Bekker figured he was as good, but not many, including his wife, saw it that way. He was a bit of a disaster on the hill, and moguls completely threw him off track. He'd even sustained a back injury one year from falling sideways when he couldn't maintain his balance on a particularly steep mogul run.

The twins could ski but preferred snowboarding on these vacations, and they liked breaking away when they could for spa sessions—that they, of course, charged to their room. Dr. Bekker never reprimanded them much, as he figured it was the price to pay for teenage daughters. Their son wasn't joining them this year, as he intended to stay behind to study for final exams. Law school was a serious plan, so his son knew it was time to buckle down and get serious about making that goal a reality.

The Bekkers prepaid the hotel they were staying at. They were using some Air Miles collected on previous trips, though Dr. Bekker didn't always remember to give them his number when they checked their luggage. His wife had created a budget for the trip—or at least set a target—and Dr. Bekker hoped they could stay within it.

In the days leading up to their trip, the Bekkers checked up on snow conditions in Whistler, and they were better than could reasonably be expected for the time of year. Thankfully, even though it was late spring, they hadn't entirely missed the season's skiing. The Bekkers arrived at the Chateau Fairmont at dinnertime and were distressed when they found out that the weather reports called for freezing rain overnight. They cursed their luck, but by morning things had cleared and they would be hitting the hills after all. The freezing rain hadn't been quite as bad as expected.

Trish Bekker preferred the challenge of the expert hills, and so did Dr. Bekker—he felt like he was getting his money's worth there. He figured they could have stayed a lot closer to home if they were prepared to settle for less. When the Bekkers started down the expert hill, they realized the conditions weren't as good as they had been led to believe. In fact, they were treacherous. Trish could manage the conditions and was skiing about five seconds ahead of him—in his line of sight. He preferred this arrangement, and it helped him on the tougher hills. But Mrs. Bekker unexpectedly hit a patch of sheer ice and took a terrible fall, sliding down the hill, skis and poles flying from under her and landing metres away from her reach.

Dr. Bekker's heart raced. He lost sight of her for a moment and then felt the ice under his skis. He dropped to his side and dug in his edges—it seemed like fifty metres, maybe more, that he'd slid out of control. He could see his wife was down and unconscious.

He ran over to her and then called 911. Mrs. Bekker was airlifted off the mountain twenty minutes later. Dr. Bekker was in a panic. He wasn't allowed on the helicopter with Trish, so he scrambled to find the twins and finally found them in the spa. Together, they drove to the hospital, where they waited for several hours without so much as a word from a nurse. Thankfully, though, his wife suffered only a concussion, lacerations to her face and upper body, torn ligaments in her right knee, and a broken tibia. "It could have been worse," Dr. Bekker would later tell people when he recounted the story.

He called his office to inform the staff of his wife's accident. The hygienists did what they could in Mrs. Bekker's absence—they rescheduled appointments and called other patients who were on Dr. Bekker's calendar for the upcoming week. One of the hygienists recorded a message, referring all regular patients with dental emergencies to one of Dr. Bekker's colleagues. The practice wasn't running efficiently, but at least patients were being taken care of and not left in the lurch.

Mrs. Bekker remained in hospital for several days before being transferred to a Vancouver hospital for reconstructive knee surgery. Dr. Bekker had no idea how long it'd take before she was well enough to fly home. It first looked like his stay with his wife would last a day or two, but that stretched into three and then four and then more days. He worried about the inconvenience and about the long-term impact on his practice.

Dr. Bekker booked a red-eye flight home a week after his wife checked into hospital; because of a lung injury, she had to wait even longer before making the trip home. Though he was in the air at midnight and was exhausted, Dr. Bekker couldn't sleep. His mind raced. He'd been a firm believer in *everything will turn out all right*, and he felt foolish because he'd never anticipated anything like this ever happening. He'd be going home alone, and he had to look after his daughters and manage his practice without his wife, who happened to handle the bills and everything else he didn't because he was busy providing care to patients. He had no idea where or how to start when he got home.

At some point over the Rockies, he thought, *It could have been worse* and *It could have been me*. He even thought, *It should have been me* because his wife was a far better skier than he was. And the more he thought about it, the more he became convinced that something like this was bound to happen to him sometime. Not skiing necessarily, but it could be an accident at home or on the road, or an illness. He felt like the odds were catching up to him and realized he had to be more responsible and plan for such unfortunate uncertainties. The situation had completely altered his perspective on how he was handling his affairs, and he gave himself a failing grade. But do better he would, he assured himself.

Dr. Bekker looked through his wallet, searching for the business card given by one of the surgeons who would be examining his wife the next day. In looking for that card, Dr. Bekker came upon another: Dr. Malhotra's. It suddenly occurred to him that the young dentist who'd given him a boost last year, the one who'd sat down with him for coffee at the conference just a week before, was certainly better equipped to handle a predicament like this one.

He put Dr. Malhotra's card in a fold in his wallet where he'd find it easily the next morning, when he'd make the call to ask about the Leighton team. It was time to get things in order.

Chapter 12: Changing course

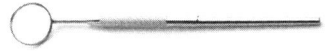

Dr. Bekker held the door open for his wife. She still found the crutches awkward, but was getting more used to them as the days went by. It had only been a week since her return home from Vancouver, and she was glad to be back.

Dr. Bekker waited until she was back before booking a meeting with Paul Leighton. Dr. Bekker called Dr. Malhotra to get the contact information, then contacted Paul right away. He told Paul that Dr. Malhotra highly recommended the group's services and asked what information and documents would be needed for a consultation. It was then that Dr. Bekker more deeply appreciated how crucial his wife was to his home life as well as the practice. She directed him to the location of various files where documents were stored and told him where to find the necessary information. The entire experience was humbling.

Paul Leighton showed the Bekkers into the conference room and found a footrest for Mrs. Bekker to rest her leg on. A few newsletters were at one end of the table—items left behind from an earlier staff meeting.

"I think I recognize those," Dr. Bekker commented.

"Oh, our newsletters? We send those out to dentists across the province," Paul said. "Our newsletters are about keeping more of what you earn in your pocket. They include tips, case studies, and tax planning advice. As Dr. Malhotra may have indicated, we structure the business affairs of our clients so they can achieve their personal objectives."

Upon further reflection, Dr. Bekker had seen those magazines at his office before but had never really given them much thought. Mrs. Bekker leafed through them as well. She at least had thought about following up on them but had put it off. The idea of a whole new round of paperwork was daunting, and even though she'd never been quite as assured as her husband was with the idea that everything would turn out fine, she was, admittedly, comfortable with the status quo.

"Trish, how are you feeling? How's the recovery process going? Dennis filled me in about what happened when he called to make this appointment."

Mrs. Bekker gave him the play-by-play and finished by saying, "I'm just glad I'm home and getting better, and that it wasn't both of us who sustained injuries. That would've been a catastrophe."

Neither of the Bekkers mentioned that the accident had played a significant role in their decision to contact the Leighton team.

Just as Paul had done with Dr. Malhotra, he told the Bekkers about his personal background and the services the Leighton team offered. "I also like to know a bit more about my clients before getting started. Why don't you give me a rundown on your life together? It'll help us out as we put together a plan for you."

"Well, we met skiing. It was in university, and the trip had been organized by the students' association. We met on the bus and talked all the way to Blue Mountain," Mrs. Bekker said.

This drew rueful laughs out of the Bekkers, but it was the truth. Mrs. Bekker was the accomplished skier while Dr. Bekker was a novice who borrowed equipment and went down the mountain like a halfback with the end zone in his sights. That was to be expected—Dr. Bekker had spent a lot more time on the football field than on the slopes, and he dove into everything with a confidence that sometimes bordered on recklessness.

The Bekkers' parents were alumni of the University of Toronto, and every child in their respective families was destined for university. Their brothers and sisters had graduated and were professionals (except possibly Mrs. Bekker's younger and somewhat Bohemiam brother, who aspired to be a visual artist). Though the Bekkers and their siblings had attended public schools, they wanted private school educations for their children—their son had gone to Upper Canada College, while their twin daughters were in their last year at Havergal.

"That's a huge financial commitment," Paul said, taking note.

"You're not kidding! What a chunk of money. When I tell them that I'm giving them a million-dollar education, it's closer to the truth than they know," Dr. Bekker said. "Fact is, when they head off to university, it's about a wash with what I've been paying so far."

"Well, that's why you're here, so we can get your money working for you." Paul outlined the services that the Leighton team could offer them. "Do you have the personal financial information form that I sent along a few days ago?"

Mrs. Bekker pulled it out from a file folder she had on her lap. "We do. It wasn't an enjoyable experience!"

Before he gave it a quick once-over, he passed Dr. and Mrs. Bekker writing paper and pens. He asked them to draw up a list of their priorities, exactly what type of help that the Leighton team could provide them. Their lists turned out more or less the same.

- *Pay less tax*
- *Better cash flow*
- *Fund children's eduction*
- *Pay down our debt*
- *Security in case of death or disability*
- *Increase retirement savings*

"Are you incorporated?" he asked. "Did your accountant ever discuss this with you?"

Dr. Bekker responded, "Well, no, I haven't incorporated. Our accountant said it might be worth considering, but we never took it beyond that."

"Are most dentists incorporated?" Mrs. Bekker asked.

"Well, all of ours are," Paul said. "Really, though, we see quite a few dentists who aren't—including many whose practices are as well-established as yours. Don't think of yourselves as an exception."

"

The primary advantage of incorporation is tax reduction.

"

Paul Leighton laid out the primary advantage of incorporation for the Bekkers—tax reduction. He said that they would be able to put aside some of their revenue that the taxman "couldn't get a bite of." He also explained how an incorporated practice could pay out dividends, and how the tax rate on those dividends could be much less than what the Bekkers paid as salaries, particularly when paid to shareholders with low income.

"You say that you have three children and one is in university," Paul said, looking at the document.

> "
>
> *The tax rate on dividends can be much less than salaries, particularly when paid to shareholders with low income.*
>
> "

"It's going to be three in university next September," said Mrs. Bekker. "Our son has completed his second year, and the twins are waiting to hear back on their applications, but they'll be going somewhere. If they have their way, it'll be Vancouver and Calgary."

Dr. Bekker was about to make a wisecrack. In other circumstances, he'd noted that he and his wife had originally planned to have only two kids. The punchline always got his wife's dander up: "Even those plans we couldn't get right." He'd received enough cold looks over the years to know that the safe line with twins was "doubly blessed."

"Twins," Paul said. "I have another client who has college-aged twins. So let me ask . . . have the twins turned eighteen yet?"

Dr. Bekker could field this question because, with his wife on the sidelines recovering from surgery, he was in charge of picking up the birthday gifts: iPads. They'd be useful in university, he was certain.

"They turn eighteen next month," he said.

"Well, incorporation can really help out with the expenses of university tuitions," Paul told the Bekkers. "As a dentist in Ontario, you can name your children as non-voting shareholders in your incorporated practice. They must be at least age eighteen. Based on today's tax rates, the dividends that you pay out to them will be essentially tax-free, up to $40,000 per year, so long as they have no other income. But that tax-free amount could well be greater than $40,000 once we consider each of their tuition credits."

"

As a dentist in Ontario, you can name your children as non-voting shareholders in your incorporated practice. They must be at least age eighteen.

"

Dr. Bekker grimaced. "You mean we could have done this with our son before he headed off to university?" he asked.

"You could have done just that," Paul told him. "But don't worry. We can set him up, along with your daughters, when we create the incorporated practice. The tax savings from dividends will work down the expenses of his education going forward."

"This is really good news, Paul," said Dr. Bekker.

"I have to agree with my husband," said Mrs. Bekker, leaning over to adjust her leg. Dr. Bekker got out of his chair to assist her.

Paul continued. "Now that I know more about your background, let's take a closer look at what's going on."

"

Adult shareholders may receive dividends up to $40,000 per year essentially tax-free provided they have no other sources of income. This amount can be higher once tuition tax credits are considered.

"

Chapter 13: The numbers

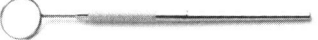

Paul pored over the financial information provided by the Bekkers, particularly their net worth and financial statements for the dental practice.

Dr. Bekker's practice seemed to provide him with a sturdy financial foundation, enough that he could provide three kids with top-notch educations, take regular family vacations, drive a luxury automobile, own a cottage in Muskoka, and live in a rather upscale part of Toronto.

The Toronto real estate market had been on a roller-coaster ride, so the Bekkers weren't sure whether they had guessed low when they'd estimated the value of their North Toronto home. They'd made an even bigger guess about their cottage in Muskoka. They really didn't keep track of the market too closely, although they knew down to the dollar what was left on the cottage's mortgage.

The Bekkers had managed to put away some money in retirement savings, but by their own admission, contributions were sporadic. They had some RRSPs, but no other savings. Paul mentally noted that some of his long-standing and more cautious clients in similar positions had close to twice the amount in their RRSPs than the Bekkers did.

The practice certainly grossed a good income, but expenses were high. The remaining net income was less than half of what it brought in, and this was before remuneration to the Bekker family. Fortunately, there was no debt within the practice because most of the major dental equipment and office furnishings had been paid for in recent years.

"These practice numbers are consistent with what I've seen with other dentists in your demographic, so you're on par, which is good," said Paul. "Based on my initial observation, we need to focus on reducing your taxes and improving your cash flow so that you can pay down your personal debt faster, save more for retirement, and cover the kid's education costs."

In total, the Bekkers were servicing $675,000 in personal debt, or almost three-quarters of a million dollars. This had never particularly concerned Dr. Bekker—at least, until his wife's injury. The Bekkers had fallen into the habit of spending all that they made. It wasn't until the practice had ground to an unexpected halt because of his wife's injuries that Dr. Bekker really had given the debt much thought.

"I know that there's a lot coming out of my practice to fund our lifestyle—the mortgages have to be paid, there's maintenance of two properties, tuition fees for all three kids, riding school fees for the twins—it seems we spend everything we bring in. Then we have to consider the added expense that came with Trish's accident: the cost of an air ambulance, a private room, a hotel room, and two tickets on short notice back to Toronto. I know what needs to be paid and what things we're paying for, but . . . ." said Dr. Bekker, stopping mid-sentence. He needed a glass of water.

"Do you want one, Trish?" She declined.

"I'm pleased that you at least know what's at stake and what needs to be considered," said Paul. "With all the meters running and the practice's income slowing dramatically because of Trish's accident, that doesn't leave much breathing room, even in the short term.

"Your biggest problems are debt and cash flow," he continued. He did a workup in pencil to give them a sense of a strategy going forward.

> *Incorporation can limit the impact of taxation on your income.*

"Let me show you in rough form how incorporation can limit the impact of taxation on your income based on the numbers you've provided me. These are what I see as the keys to our strategy for your situation. We want to pay down your debt, we want to put money aside for your retirement, and we want to put you in the best position to look after your children's education, which is relatively simple to do."

Paul moved his chair to sit closer to Dr. and Mrs. Bekker. "If you look here, this is an example of what we could do if you incorporated," he said, and he started writing. "We'll assume that the practice's gross income and business expenses stay the same, but now you, Dennis, draw a salary. Now you can make maximum contributions to an RRSP or an Individual Pension Plan (IPP). I'm thinking that an IPP may be the preferred retirement savings structure for you both because it offers larger deductions than RRSPs for those over the age of forty."

Dr. Bekker rubbed his forehead in an effort to concentrate. This was out of his realm, but he knew he had to understand it so he could be a part of the decision making. Paul continued with his calculations.

> *The bottom line is that incorporation can reduce taxes by thousands, perhaps tens of thousands per year.*

"Trish, you could continue to draw a salary for management of the office, just as you do now, keeping you in a lower tax bracket than Dennis. It's a reasonable salary given your duties in the practice. After you both draw your salaries and make annual IPP contributions, you'll have to pay corporate tax on what remains in the company. The amount that's left can be paid to family members in the form of tax-free dividends from the profit.

"The bottom line," Paul said, "is that we can reduce your taxes by thousands, perhaps tens of thousands per year."

"Wow," said Dr. Bekker. "By all means, let's see if we can make this happen!"

They agreed that Paul would draw up exactly how incorporation would look for Dr. Bekker's practice. He then asked them to spend a few days assessing their financial needs to sustain a lifestyle that they were comfortable with. "And if the budget isn't realistic, no financial planning will have much of a chance to be a long-term success. Draw up numbers based on your current personal spending habits and estimate the children's university costs."

> *If the budget isn't realistic, no financial planning will have much of a chance to be a long-term success.*

The Bekkers nodded, but they assumed there'd still be some hardship involved in covering their kids' education. Paul believed he could make that financially painless. And he would, in fact, pull it off.

Chapter 14: Ready for change

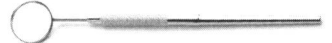

It occurred to Dr. Bekker that he might have tuned out any financial pep talk like Paul Leighton's at an earlier point in his life. He'd grown up in middle-class Leaside; his parents were a successful real estate team. They weren't members of the Granite Club, but they'd made sure their kids wanted for nothing.

Dr. Bekker was the family star—the best athlete, the best student, and the one who'd picked things up more quickly than others in dental school. He saw friends who, no matter how hard they worked, weren't destined to graduate. He didn't think of himself as exceptional, even if they did. Still, early on he knew he'd have a successful practice.

Now Dr. Bekker felt somewhat vulnerable. He'd gained a whole new perspective on his career, which had so far offered him a chance for security and a good lifestyle, but hadn't yet offered him any guarantees. After dinner that night, a few hours after seeing Paul, Dr. Bekker and his wife stayed at the dinner table. With them they had a drawer's worth of receipts and a pen and pad of paper. They started determining what their lifestyle consisted of and what they truly felt they needed to live comfortably.

First they recorded their mortgages, taxes, and insurance payments on their properties. They figured out their regular household expenses: groceries (sure to be reduced with their children at school), their weekly housecleaning service, seasonal gardening, and miscellaneous and sundry items. Then there was insurance on their vehicles (having three young drivers in the house drove the premium through the roof) and gas, which always seemed to be going up in price. Dr. Bekker allotted an amount for servicing of the vehicles but knew that it was low, or at least optimistic, with the warrantees expiring.

"

Determine what your lifestyle consists of and what you truly feel you need to live comfortably.

"

They also added in personal life and disability premiums and agreed to maximize their RRSP contributions each year.

After looking up the costs of tuition, room and board and estimating books, electronics, and travel, they put down the costs of the kids' education.

As per Paul's advice, the Bekkers tried to be comprehensive and realistic. They had never before felt guilty about their spending habits, and they didn't now, which is why they weren't going to let some things go. After reviewing their various credit card statements, they put down an honest amount for clothing and other discretionary expenses (dining out, vacations, kids' activities, and general spending money).

"I have a suggestion, Trish. Let's track our finances over the course of the year, starting next month. If we start to exceed our budget, let's rent the cottage out for a week or two, or possibly more in late summer."

"Dennis, we've talked about this before, and I quite like the idea. There are weeks when the cottage is empty, and you dread the crush of vacationers on Highway 11 and the 401 on Labour Day weekend. This process really has us looking at the value we're getting, or not, on what we spend, and the cottage is definitely something we aren't capitalizing on. Why don't we wait a few months, assess our progress, then determine whether the rental would be necessary or useful."

"Good thinking, Trish. Do you want that last piece of pie?"

The Bekkers worked down the list item by item. After one hour, they settled on a total of $240,000 to cover personal expenses, education, and savings. Whether it was a well-considered projection or a guesstimate didn't matter to Dr. Bekker—he swore he could feel his belt pinching his waistline (or was that the two pieces of blueberry pie he'd just eaten?).

Chapter 15: Passing the budget

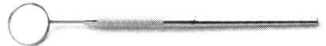

At the next meeting, the Bekkers gave their budget to Paul and explained how they'd arrived at the numbers. They detailed how the cottage rental could give them a margin for error.

"These are numbers I can work with," Paul said. "But I have to know you can make a commitment to keep within these expenses."

"We've thought about it long and hard, and we can be more committed," said Mrs. Bekker, lightly patting her husband's hand.

"Give me a couple of minutes to review these numbers and see if we can make this work for you," Paul said. While he worked quietly, the Bekkers got up and helped themselves to a glass of water.

Paul created two number columns on a blank sheet of paper. After a few minutes, he took another sheet and wrote in numbers large enough that they could be seen across the conference table.

"Okay, I'm ready. Without incorporation, you'd normally pay $120,000 in taxes. But under the plan I'm proposing, the total tax bill, personal and corporate combined, drops to $76,500, which is $43,500 in tax savings per year."

The Bekkers stared at the page in wonder. "This is remarkable," Dr. Bekker heard himself say. "How is this possible?"

"It's the power of income splitting. Dennis, you might recall a few years ago that the provincial college of dentists and the provincial government decided to allow dentists to incorporate, but they also allowed family members to become non-voting shareholders. Because your children currently have no other sources of income, they can receive a lot of dividend income from your company without paying personal income tax.

> *An Individual Pension Plan (IPP) is the preferred retirement savings structure for those over forty because it allows the ability to save for retirement faster.*

"Your annual savings in income taxes available through incorporation," Paul reiterated, "is money you'll have available that you otherwise wouldn't if you were to remain unincorporated—presuming there are no substantial changes in the net income and expenses in your practice.

"The basics stay the same with respect to your revenue and expenses. The only difference is that I suggest you start an Individual Pension Plan instead of RRSPs because an IPP allows you to save for retirement faster. As you'll see below, IPP contributions are a corporate deduction, unlike RRSPs, which are a personal deduction."

Paul showed them the next page he'd written up. "This is how it all looks. Let's take a minute to review it together."

Paul then explained how, once incorporated, Dr. Bekker's practice could contribute to his retirement plan through an IPP, a move that would accelerate his retirement savings. He also outlined how dividends would be paid equally, and tax-free, to each of his kids, which would help pay for their education.

He also explained, "If not all the money is needed toward your children's education, you can dedicate some of that money to reducing debt. And when they finish their education, you'll have some other options available because when they start their careers and generate their own incomes, those dividends will be taxed more heavily. Then you'd be looking at other ways to make your money work for you."

"At the very bottom line," Paul explained, "the combined salaries and dividends from the incorporated practice leaves *more after-tax* than the net income from your unincorporated practice. Incorporation simply makes sense in your situation." In a matter of minutes, Paul had shown them how to dramatically improve their cash flow and reduce their taxes.

"

By reducing your tax bill, you could accomplish so much more in your financial life.

"

After some additional calculations, it meant that the Bekkers would have $29,550 per year left that they could direct toward their own lifestyle expenses or paying down debts faster.

"At this pace," Paul remarked, "You could be debt free by retirement."

Despite all the number juggling, the Bekkers were still following Paul's explanation. By reducing their tax bill, they could accomplish so much more in their financial lives. They could afford to put *all* their kids through university without having to work longer hours and make sacrifices. They could knock down their debt and save toward their retirement faster. And it'd mean they could sleep better at night.

"Paul, this is outstanding. I'm eager to hear what other steps we can take to further improve our finances. Are there other things we can do, or is this it?" Dr. Bekker asked hesitantly.

"There are! We need to further discuss the idea of incorporation, which is key to many of these things working," said Paul.

As he had with Dr. Malhotra, Paul explained to the Bekkers the fundamentals involved with setting up the practice as a corporation. It was complex, given that Dr. Bekker had an established practice with staff, equipment, and a premises lease, not to mention the need for multiple classes of shares.

"

During the incorporation process, there's an opportunity to transfer your business assets to the Professional Corporation, such as equipment and leaseholds. Because these have already been purchased with after-tax dollars, you can withdraw the same amount from your company tax-free later on.

"

"During the incorporation process, there's an opportunity to transfer your business assets to the Professional Corporation, such as equipment and leaseholds. Because these have already been purchased with after-tax dollars, you can withdraw the same amount from your company tax-free later on. This is called a 'roll over' in tax terms. And if the money isn't readily available, it could be borrowed from the operating line of credit. This money could be used to pay off personal non-deductible debts, such as your mortgage. Effectively, we'd be able to convert a non-deductible debt into a tax-deductible debt." Dr. and Mrs. Bekker began nodding in appreciation and understanding. Paul continued.

"

Wills and powers of attorney are such important documents in your overall estate plan that they need to get done properly.

"

"Aside from how incorporation can improve your bottom line and cash flow, we need to address something equally important—managing your risk. Let me ask you something, have you had your wills and powers of attorney prepared?"

Dr. Bekker looked at Mrs. Bekker, who shook her head. "No, not yet," said Dr. Bekker rather sheepishly.

"Well, you're not the only ones to respond that way. Many people I speak with haven't had them completed," Paul said. "These are such important documents in your overall estate plan that they need to get done right. Wills can actually save you money, too. With use of a secondary will, you can save the probate fees on the shares of your Professional Corporation. Given the value of your dental practice, I'd estimate about $12,000. Not too bad for the nominal cost of a second will."

> *With use of a secondary will, you can save the probate fees on the shares of your Professional Corporation.*

"Can you recommend someone?" asked Mrs. Bekker.

"Of course, absolutely. I'll introduce you to a lawyer who's experienced in estate planning, but I'll stay on top of you to ensure it gets done," Paul gently suggested. "The other way we manage risk is to ensure you're properly insured, and not just with life insurance. Life insurance is important, but it's not the only risk to manage. At your age, it's more likely you'll be injured for an extended period of time," Paul said, as he glanced briefly at Mrs. Bekker's leg, which was still in a cast, "or that you develop a critical illness, such as cancer, or suffer heart attack or stroke, all things that would prevent you from working for a while. We need to consider these contingencies to ensure you can still manage things comfortably should one of these occur."

Dr. Bekker explained he had life insurance policies as required to cover the debts on their properties, with a bit extra to replace lost income for the survivor. Dr. Bekker also had disability insurance he'd taken out years before, when he started practicing dentistry.

Paul pointed out the deficiency in their life insurance coverage in order to provide a greater amount of replacement income, and to ensure the children's education expenses would be covered. Term insurance would be sufficient because the need was of a temporary nature, perhaps the next ten years. In addition, term insurance would be available at the most affordable rates compared to other types of plans. Permanent life insurance, such as whole life or universal life, could be considered at a later date once their debts were paid off and retirement savings built up, Paul noted.

For the first time, though, Dr. Bekker gave thought to backup plans that they didn't have in place—namely, long-term disability for his wife and critical illness insurance for them both.

"We see now how quickly our health can change and the impact it can have on our finances. Our eyes are wide open, and thankfully it's nothing as debilitating or critical as cancer. We can get through this and we're just glad we have a chance to start over and make things right," said Dr. Bekker.

"Without a doubt, Dennis. It's not too late to turn things around. I suggest that life policies be owned and paid by your company. It's a more efficient use of your cash flow. Because the corporate tax rate is less than your personal tax rate, there's more money left over to pay the insurance premium. While the cost isn't tax-deductible, the death benefit remains tax-free to the company, and in many situations, can be paid tax-free to the surviving shareholders. Disability and critical illness plans should continue to be paid personally. Otherwise, the benefits would be taxable."

After addressing the issues of incorporation and risk management, Paul turned his attention back to the Bekkers' debt and cash flow. Cash flow was a critically important element in helping understand each client's unique circumstances. Paul often thought it was like the initial examination that a patient had with a dentist—it was necessary to understand the current situation before making specific recommendations.

"The overhead expense on your practice is 60 percent; that leaves 40 percent available as compensation for you and your family. That's not bad, but there's definitely room for improvement in efficiency. Practices can aim for, and achieve, a 50:50 split on expenses and practice profits with some adjustments in management," Paul said. "We've even had some clients reduce their expenses below 50 percent of the practice profits.

"In your case, if we're presuming that your net income and your compensation remains the same, a drop to a 50:50 ratio of expenses to profits would net you better than $76,000 a year."

The Bekkers nodded, understanding what Paul was saying. They had never considered these things before, but were completely getting the big picture now that Paul was walking them through it.

"An extra $76,000 after tax," Paul said. "That sounds like a lot just on the face of it. The effect of that extra income can have a huge impact on your ability to build your corporate savings, and ultimately, your retirement nest egg. Let's use your practice revenue and expenses to show how savings can accumulate in your corporation."

He quickly tabulated the numbers on his financial calculator, wrote them down, and then showed them to the Bekkers.

Ratio of Expenses to Revenue	@ 70:30	@ 60:40	@50:50
Gross Revenue	$900,000	$900,000	$900,000
Operating Expenses	($630,000)	($540,000)	($450,000)
Family Salaries	($199,200)	($199,200)	($199,200)
IPP	($47,200)	($47,200)	($47,200)
Income	$23,600	$113,600	$203,600
Corporate Taxes	($3,600)	($17,600)	($31,600)
Net Income	**$20,000**	**$96,000**	**$172,000**
6% Annual Return after 15 Years	**$493,000**	**$2,368,000**	**$4,243,000**

"An efficient practice can help achieve your retirement goals faster. You can see how quickly those dollars accumulate," Paul said. "Now those numbers aren't quite what you'd be looking at, in part because of your intention to pay out dividends to your children while they're in school. But in a few years, when they're starting their careers, they won't be drawing out significant dividends—there'll be no advantage for them. At that point, you can redirect the surplus profits toward investments for your retirement goals."

The Bekkers made a mental note of this, knowing how quickly time passed. "Paul, later on can we discuss areas where we might rein in our expenses?" asked Mrs. Bekker.

"We have a practice management expert that can give you some advice and help you tweak things," Paul replied. "But typically you'd start with the largest expenses. Based on our observations, the biggest expenses are staff, supplies, lab, and rent. If you can make improvements in these areas, you'll definitely maximize your savings."

Dr. Bekker jumped in. "I have some concerns, particularly the long-term lease on the office. It expires next year, and frankly, I've been unhappy with the terms. I didn't like the numbers last time, but I felt worn down and decided to sign to get it over with," he told Paul. "I'd like to look at some other options, whether it's a move or renegotiation."

"I can refer you to lawyers with expertise in this area, as well as commercial real estate brokers who know what rents are being paid by dentists with practices on your scale. I'll e-mail you some names later in the week."

"Thanks very much," said Dr. Bekker, who made a note of it on his file folder.

"Well, that about wraps it up for today. We covered an enormous amount of ground. At another visit, I'd recommend we look at some retirement projections and investment strategies, to address your long-term goals. Do you have any questions, concerns?"

"No, none. We'll need to go home and digest everything you told us, but I think I speak for both of us when I say that we're far more hopeful about our financial prospects than when we arrived," said Dr. Bekker, looking over at Mrs. Bekker, who nodded in complete agreement.

Chapter 16: What they decided

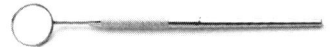

On the way home after their meeting, the Bekkers reflected on how they had handled their finances prior to Trish's skiing accident. They'd always assumed that if the office was handled well, the finances would look after themselves. As long as there were patients making appointments, the cash flow would be there and they would be able to make it work—it was how they'd operated for twenty years.

They realized now that they needed guidance from someone who could provide a coordinated approach to their finances. The next day, they contacted Paul Leighton to take the next steps together.

Given their desire to set their finances on the right path in many different areas, they opted for the Leighton team's Comprehensive Plan. The plan included:

- *coordinating the task of incorporating of Dr. Bekker's practice and setting up shareholders*

- *annual tax planning, such as determining the optimal salary/dividend mix between all family members*
- *preparing corporate financial statements and tax returns*
- *bookkeeping*
- *preparing personal tax returns for all family members*
- *assistance in implementing their personal financial plan, such as retirement planning, investment advice, estate planning and rewriting their wills, insurance planning, and debt management*
- *referrals to specialists with expertise in various areas, such as lawyers for business or estate planning, practice management consultants, lease renewal consultants, or practice valuators*

"

Many areas need to be tackled, such as retirement planning, investments, proper insurance coverage, and possibly debt consolidation.

"

Paul said he'd arrange for a lawyer who specialized in the incorporation of dentists to start the process right away. As he'd mentioned, many areas still needed to be tackled, such as their retirement planning, investments, proper insurance coverage, and possibly debt consolidation. These would be addressed on a continuous basis. A follow-up meeting was scheduled for the following month once the incorporation was completed.

The Bekkers were confident that this level of service would address their immediate needs and set them up for a secure and prosperous future. Given that they'd been carrying the weight of their son's university tuition and the twins' private-school education, the Bekkers expected to suffer no hardship in sticking to their budget. Incorporation made their finances not only viable but also more comfortable.

"

Incorporation makes finances not only viable but also more comfortable.

"

Chapter 17: Giving thanks for good advice

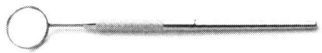

In midsummer, Dr. Bekker did a little personal housekeeping and cleaned out his wallet, which was bulging with business cards from folks he'd met on the golf course. He saw Dr. Malhotra's business card and decided to send an e-mail to the young dentist.

> *Arjun,*
>
> *I want to thank you for referring me to the Leighton team. My wife and I signed on with Paul several weeks ago. I wouldn't say that I'm a changed man or anything, but I would say that I feel a lot more confident about the future knowing my practice and finances are in control. I feel like a guy who was on a treadmill that kept churning faster and faster . . . not that I got off that treadmill or that I stopped it, but at least now it's going at a speed that I can manage. I hope to see you at a conference or perhaps a trade event.*
>
> *Dennis*

Dr. Malhotra replied to Dr. Bekker right away.

Dennis,

I'm glad things are working out for you. I can only say that I hope one day to have a practice as well established as yours and a family that does so well. I look forward to seeing you again. If I'm in Toronto I'll drop you a line, and if you're ever up in the London area, please get in touch.

Arjun

Dr. Dennis Bekker, DDS

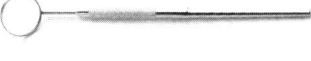

Mature Dentist

- 50 years old

- Graduated 22 years ago from the Faculty of Dentistry, University of Toronto

- Dental practice located in Toronto

- Married to Trish Bekker, who works as office manager in Dr. Bekker's practice

- Three children: Clayton (20), twins Tracey and Anna (17)

Dr. Bekker had handicapped himself for years by not having a cohesive financial plan. Finally he had one. Here's what it looked like.

Goals

- Reduce taxes
- Improve cash flow
- Fund children's education
- Pay down debt
- Security in case of death or disability
- Retirement

Cash Flow

INCOME

Practice Revenue	$900,000
Expenses (@ 60% of revenue)	($540,000)
Salary to Mrs. Bekker	($72,000)
Personal Income to Dr. Bekker	$288,000
Salary to Mrs. Bekker	$72,000
Personal Tax & CPP (combined or both spouses)	($120,000)
Net cash flow	**$240,000**

LIFESTYLE EXPENSES

Home and vacation property	$72,000
Food and other household expenses	$24,550
Automobile expenses	$14,000
Personal discretionary spending	$25,000
Life and disability insurance	$9,000
Education expenses for 3 children	$60,000
RRSP contributions	$35,450
Total annual spending	**$240,000**

Net Worth

ASSETS

Home	$850,000
Vacation Property	$500,000
Vehicles	$75,000
Registered Retirement Savings Plan (RRSP)	$305,000
Dental Practice	$800,000
	$2,530,000

LIABILITIES

Mortgage	$400,000
Vacation Property	$275,000
	$675,000

NET WORTH   **$1,855,000**

Incorporation, Tax Reduction & Cash Flow Improvement

Establish a Professional Corporation, with Dr. Bekker as voting shareholder, and his spouse and three kids as non-voting shareholders. Dr. Bekker & Mrs. Bekker will own "growth" shares to avail themselves of the $750,000 capital gains deduction.

	Sole Proprietor	Incorporated
Revenue	$900,000	$900,000
Expenses (@ 60% of revenue)	($540,000)	($540,000)
Salary to Dr. Bekker		($125,000)
Employer CPP (Dr. Bekker)		($2,200)
Salary to Mrs. Bekker	($72,000)	($72,000)
IPP Contributions		($47,200)
Corporate net income		$113,600
Corporate taxes		($17,600)
Corporate income after tax		$96,000
Personal Income to Dr. Bekker	$288,000	$125,000
Salary to Mrs. Bekker	$72,000	$72,000
Personal Tax & CPP	($120,000)	($58,900)
Net cash flow	**$240,000**	**$234,100**
Lifestyle needs (as above)	($144,550)	($144,550)
Education expenses	($60,000)	($60,000)
RRSP contributions	($35,450)	$0
Additional debt repayment	**$0**	**$29,550**
Total Taxes	**$120,000**	**$76,500**
TAX REDUCTION / CASH FLOW IMPROVEMENT		**$43,500**

Total taxes are reduced by $43,500 per year and cash flow increased.

Incorporation, Tax Reduction & Cash Flow Improvement (continued)

Prior to incorporation, Dr. Bekker's net income was $288,000. Both spouses contributed maximum RRSPs.

After incorporation, Dr. Bekker's earned a salary of $125,000. The company contributed towards IPPs on behalf of both spouses. Remaining corporate profits paid as dividends to children.

Personal taxes reduced from $120,000 to $58,900.

	Dr Bekker	Mrs Bekker	(3) Children	Total Tax
Before Incorporation				
Salary / Professional Income	$288,000	$72,000	$0	
Dividends	$0	$0	$0	
RRSP	$22,450	$13,000	$0	
Personal Tax	$101,500	$11,900	$0	$113,400
CPP	$4,400	$2,200	$0	$6,600
Total Personal Tax & CPP	$105,900	$14,100	$0	$120,000
After Incorporation				
Salary / Professional Income	$125,000	$72,000	$0	
Dividends	$0	$0	$96,000	
RRSP	$0	$0	$0	
Personal Tax	$37,150	$16,000	$1,350*	$54,500
CPP	$2,200	$2,200	$0	$4,400
Total Personal Tax & CPP	$39,350	$18,200	$1,350	$58,900

* Ontario Health Premium is the only tax attributable to the children.

Children's Education Funding

Without incorporation, the children's education costs of $60,000 per year were to be paid with personal cash flow. Dr. Bekker would need to earn $112,000 before tax to cover these costs (top marginal tax rate of 46.4%).

After incorporation and adding children as shareholders, the children could receive $60,000 of dividends with very little tax. The Professional Corporation would need to earn $71,000 before tax to cover these costs (at the small business tax rate of 15.5%).

As a result, the Bekker's saved taxes of $41,000 per year by paying dividends to their children to cover education costs.

Debt Repayment

Transfer dental assets ($50,000) into the practice, then take back tax-free shareholder advance to help reduce personal debt.

	Current	Proposed
Mortgage	$400,000	$400,000
Vacation Property	$275,000	$275,000
Less: Shareholder Advance		($50,000)
Total Liabilities	$675,000	$625,000
Normal Mortgage Payments [1]	$49,000	$49,000
Prepayments from Dividends	$0	$29,550
# Years to Pay-off Debt	20 Years	10 Years

With proposed restructuring, debt can be paid off 10 years sooner.

[1] Based on 20-year amortization @ 4% interest, compounded semi-annually.

Insurance Highlights

- Dr. Bekker & Mrs. Bekker to obtain enough life insurance to pay all debts, with additional coverage to replace lost income of the deceased spouse.
- Life insurance to be owned and paid by the Professional Corporation.
- Permanent life insurance, such as whole life or universal life, could be considered as an estate planning tool to offset taxes payable by their estate, or as a savings vehicle for their retirement. This could be started at a later date once the children's education expenses stopped.
- Disability and Critical illness policies to be owned and paid personally.

Retirement Planning

At a future meeting, Leighton and the Bekker's to discuss retirement plans and investment strategy.

A target retirement goal and sources of income to be determined, based on projected lifestyle spending, and current and future savings.

Investment Strategy to include:

- Investment Policy Statement (IPS)
- Low-cost, index-type investment solution
- Asset allocation to cushion market volatility
- Global diversification to balance market exposure around the world
- Tax efficiency to minimize tax paid on investment income
- Costs & tax deductibility of fees to minimize the cost of investing

Results

- $675,000 of debt paid off 10 years sooner with reduced taxes and increased cash flow

- Tax-free dividends of $60,000 annually paid for children's eduction costs

Results (continued)

- Corporate investments and Individual Pension Plan (IPP) boosts retirement income

- Insurance solution to be implemented at a future meeting

- Retirement needs addressed using surplus cash now available in the corporation guided by prudent investment strategies

Section III: Dr. St. Louis' Exit Strategy

Chapter 18: Planning for retirement

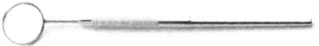

Dr. St. Louis and her husband were in a period of transition in their lives. Her husband, Professor St. Louis, was looking to teach just one class on a regular basis and to spend more time writing, creatively this time as opposed to academically. After a couple of school years more and a sabbatical year, he planned to step away from university life completely and draw on his pension, which would be a comfortable amount.

Dr. St. Louis, however, was more absolute about the change. She intended to practise up until late June, at which point Dr. Parry would take over. If she could negotiate her terms, the shares of Dr. Adeline St. Louis Dentistry Professional Corp. would be sold to Dr. Trevor Parry or his Professional Corporation. But only once their lawyers started the negotiation process would these details be discussed.

On one level, the St. Louises were easing themselves into retirement, but on another they were executing a well-laid plan based on objectives set many years earlier. There were times and places for impulses and spontaneity—they frequently changed their vacation travel plans mid-trip—but the St. Louises wanted structure and security in their professional lives and finances. In keeping with the way they both made decisions in their careers, Dr. St. Louis had given a lot of thought to their retirement years.

Dr. St. Louis had first discussed her retirement plans with Paul Leighton at her first visit with him more than fifteen years earlier, in what had been the most lucrative phase of her practice to that point.

In that first meeting, Paul had explained that many financial planners advance the notion that retirees require only 70 percent of their pre-retirement earnings to cover their projected expenses.

"

Target 100 percent of your pre-retirement lifestyle.

"

"Many people envision their retirement as a phase of life when both they and their needs slow down. However, 70 percent is, in my experience, a poor measure of a professional's retirement income needs. It doesn't seem realistic to expect someone in retirement to make a clean break from expectations and spending habits that they've developed over the course of decades," Paul had told Dr. St. Louis in that initial consultation.

"I try to steer my clients towards the target of 100 percent of their pre-retirement lifestyle. It should be a seamless transition, no reduction of means from the last day of your working career to the first day of your retirement."

At the time of her first discussion with Paul, Dr. St. Louis hadn't given much thought to a retirement savings target, but figured it was easily within reach. Her retirement was still fifteen to twenty years away, giving her ample time to build a nest egg. She estimated that she and her husband would require an annual income of $180,000 to maintain their lifestyle into retirement. Given that Professor St. Louis would receive a pension of $60,000 per year from his university if he stayed on until retirement, their savings would need to produce an additional $120,000 per year.

But when Dr. St. Louis asked Paul what she would need to sustain a personal income of $120,000 a year, she was taken aback by his answer: "It would require investable assets of $3 million to comfortably sustain a retirement income in that range," he answered. He then explained that a realistic and sustainable annual retirement income should represent 4 percent of investable assets.

"

A realistic and sustainable annual retirement income should represent 4 percent of investable assets.

"

Just as the $3 million number had seemed high to Dr. St. Louis, the 4 percent felt too low. She'd presumed that the sale of her practice prior to her retirement would cover the bulk of her needs. Paul pointed out that retirement can be "a longer time than you might imagine. At thirty years or more, it can last as long as or even longer than your working career. The sale of a practice on even the most favourable terms would only account for about one-third of the income needed from your portfolio over the long run."

> *The sale of a practice on even the most favourable terms would only account for about one-third of the income needed from your portfolio over the long run.*

This was a sobering bit of arithmetic, and it made Dr. St. Louis see the wisdom in Paul's advice.

"You have to save early and save often," Paul told her.

> *Save early and save often.*

Chapter 19: Smart investments

A lot had changed since Dr. St. Louis first visited the Leighton team's offices. Her children had graduated university, married, and had children of their own. Her practice had steadily grown until it was one of the more lucrative in the capital region. She managed to align her practice with her life with ongoing updates of the comprehensive financial plan prepared by the Leighton team. This helped coordinate her practice's cash flows, tax-reduction strategies, investments, estate plan, insurance, and the eventual practice transition before retirement. Most important of all, her net worth had soared. An outsider might have wondered if she'd been successful at playing the market, but that simply wasn't her style.

Dr. St. Louis often read the business pages but she did so for entertainment, not for advice. Although she had incurred a fee for a stock trade a few times over all those years, she'd done so for her own amusement. She certainly didn't consider herself to be an investment guru. Most importantly, regardless of what she read or heard about in the business pages, she avoided getting caught up trying to figure out or beat the market. When asked about how she made investment decisions, she'd given the same answer she'd heard from Paul so many times before: "It's not what I do, but rather what I don't do."

"

It's not what you do, but rather what you don't do.

"

Dr. St. Louis, like others among the Leighton team's clients, remained invested in the market to stay ahead of inflation and realize growth of her financial assets. None of them made an attempt to outsmart the market. There weren't any IPOs or "hot" stocks in Dr. St. Louis' portfolio—contrary to the opinion of many of her colleagues, including a few envious ones. Holding a portfolio in the market with low-cost, index-based investments suited Dr. St. Louis' nature. And as a result the markets worked for her—costs were kept low and she continued to earn returns on her investments.

Over the years, she and Paul had many discussions about the Leighton team's investment philosophy. Paul would talk about the "big three," meaning the three parts of the approach. Although Dr. St. Louis couldn't always recall every detail, she had no trouble remembering—and trusting—the main points because as the years went by, she saw the results it created for her and her husband.

Invest, don't speculate

One of the first items Dr. St. Louis had noticed on Paul's desk was a quote from John Kenneth Galbraith: "We have two classes of forecasters: those who don't know and those who don't know they don't know." Paul used this to explain the difference between index managers and active managers.

> *Invest, don't speculate.*

"Active money managers make up the majority of brokers and investment advisors on Bay Street and Wall Street," he'd told her. "They attempt to beat the market by predicting the direction of the economy and other factors, then pick the right stocks to buy and sell at the right time."

> *"We have two classes of forecasters: those who don't know and those who don't know they don't know."*

Though it surprised her at first, Paul had explained how, over time, only a small fraction of these active money managers get this right—that is, outperform the market after fees. "This is because today's markets are very efficient due to the instantaneous flow of information," Paul said. "It's therefore far better to take advantage of the collective knowledge of the best minds in the world rather than take on more cost and more risk trying to beat them."

Over the years, the Leighton team's recommended approach was passive investing, often known as indexing, because it led to proven results for their clients. As Paul told Dr. St. Louis, an index manager doesn't attempt to "beat" the market but instead invests in all stocks comprising the index, such as the Toronto Stock Exchange or the S&P 500. Paul shared the latest annual study done by Standard & Poor's, looking at the performance of active managers over the last five years. The results showed that no more than a small fraction of managers beat their respective indexes in Canada, the US, and internationally.

"

A large amount of evidence proves that, over time, passive investing provides significantly better results with lower risk than active investing.

"

Paul showed a large amount of evidence proving that, over time, passive investing provided significantly better results with lower risk than active investing. Dr. St. Louis saw that it was an approach marked by patience rather than aggression, one that would provide an investor like her with real profit generated in the real economy by real business.

Minimize the "costs of investment"

Paul told Dr. St. Louis that active investing would diminish the value of her investments over a long time period, because it causes what's known as "drag" on portfolio growth. The passive investing approach typically costs less, about 1 to 2 percent per year. These costs can be management fees, fund expenses, and additional taxes generated by capital gains.

> *Minimize the "costs of investment."*

As Paul explained, active managers tend to trade more often and more aggressively than index managers, so it's not uncommon for turnover in actively managed funds to exceed index funds. The incentive to trade more often—that is, to actively manage your funds—does not necessarily provide better investment returns. Traditionally, brokers are compensated for their services through payments or commissions from investments they select and transactions they complete. Paul stressed that fee-only advisors, such as the Leighton team, work directly for the client. Paul felt it was their fiduciary responsibility to put clients' interests first. Dr. St. Louis liked the sound of that.

Apply a disciplined, strategic approach to controlling risk

> *Apply a disciplined, strategic approach to controlling risk.*

One of the most important jobs that a financial advisor can do is to help clients control their emotional reactions to market fluctuations. Dr. St. Louis saw from experience how important this was for helping her keep a long-term perspective and sticking to her investment plan, regardless of the latest media hype or advice from well-meaning friends and relatives.

"

Keep a long-term perspective and stick to your investment plan.

"

As Paul described it, the sensational and emotionally charged headlines in print and online are designed to grab readers' attention. "Don't confuse entertainment with advice," Paul liked to remind her. "Getting emotionally involved can compromise long-term focus and discipline, and can even lead to poor investment decisions."

"

The sensational and emotionally charged headlines in print and online are designed to grab readers' attention. Don't confuse entertainment with advice.

"

The three parts of the Leighton team's disciplined and strategic approach to investing also supported their approach to risk. Dr. St. Louis had raised her concerns about risk at one of their first meetings. Paul had replied that the Leighton team believed it was important for their clients to be invested in the capital markets because this was core to a strategic approach to controlling risk. He explained about how investment in the market would preserve the after-tax purchasing power of her and her husband's savings, after adjusting for inflation.

Paul explained that one of the best ways to control risk is using the appropriate mix of liquid cash (such as money market funds, treasury bills), stocks (when a company does well, its shareholders do well and may receive dividends), and bonds (a safe tool for reducing risk). This is why they'd created a diversified portfolio for the St. Louises designed to match their risk profile and investment objectives.

Setting up retirement income

A disciplined and strategic approach to investing and controlling risk wasn't the only evidence of Dr. St. Louis' cautious approach to her finances. When considering how she'd achieve her retirement goals, she opted for the full range of tax-efficient strategies. Years ago, Dr. St. Louis had stopped contributing to her RRSP in favour of an Individual Pension Plan. Paul liked to describe the IPP as "the best-kept secret in retirement planning." A company-sponsored IPP allowed greater annual contributions than were permitted into an RRSP, particularly to a dentist in Dr. St. Louis' demographic—over forty and with a personal income of more than $125,000.

For additional tax-efficiency, Paul strategically allocated her fixed-income assets to the tax-sheltered plan, with dividend and capital gains-producing assets to the taxable investment accounts.

Starting in 2009 and each year thereafter, Dr. St. Louis also contributed the maximum amount to her Tax-Free Savings Account (TFSA). It was her piece of financial insurance—the funds that accrued in this account could be withdrawn at any time for any purpose without a tax penalty. Only once did she do this—for emergency repairs on their vacation property in Morin-Heights. But as the TFSA regulations allowed, she was able to replace all the funds that she withdrew at a later date.

As Dr. St. Louis liked to say, she was so focused on the future that she "even looked beyond retirement." It was a joke, but there was more than a thread of truth in it. Her estate planning was comprehensive. With the aid of the Leighton team's estate planning expert, Dr. St. Louis positioned her beneficiaries to the full advantage of tax laws.

"

The use of testamentary trusts has the potential to reduce taxes on investment income, and protect children in the event of a troubled marriage.

"

To this end, she and her husband had secondary wills to avoid probate fees on the shares of the Professional Corporation. In addition, she and her husband included the use of testamentary trusts in their wills for the benefit of their children. Assuming the children invested part of their inheritances, the trusts had the potential to reduce taxes on the investment income. As an additional benefit, they provided an extra level of security should one of their children find themselves in a troubled marriage, because the funds in trust wouldn't form part of the common assets to be divided with the other spouse.

In addition to their wills, Dr. St. Louis and her husband set up a corporate-owned life insurance policy to accomplish two objectives. First, the life insurance component could be used to offset the anticipated taxes payable after the death of the surviving spouse. There would be tax payable on the remainder of their IPP (just as there would be with RRSPs or Registered Retirement Income Funds [RRIFs]), plus capital gains on their vacation property and other non-registered investments. Most, if not all, of the life insurance proceeds would be paid tax-free and could be used to offset these taxes.

Second, the life policy allowed Dr. St. Louis to redirect corporate savings that were heavily taxed into a tax-sheltered investment vehicle. These funds would be available as another source of retirement income, if ever needed. She appreciated the dual nature of this insurance strategy because it addressed two important estate planning and retirement planning concerns while reducing her immediate taxes at the same time.

Dr. St. Louis' dedication to the detailed financial plan Paul had drawn up enabled her to hit her retirement targets well before her sixtieth birthday.

Chapter 20: Security within reach

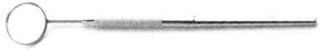

Dr. St. Louis was a model client and one of many success stories for the Leighton team. She truly believed in taking care of her financial health the same way she advised her patients to take care of their physical health—with the appropriate professionals at her side. When consulting with other dentists, Paul didn't use her name or offer any details that would give away her identity, but he did cite her retirement planning as an example of how a dentist could maximize the financial potential of an established practice in the range of $1.2 million in annual billings.

Through shrewd management of her practice's finances, and following the advice of Paul, Dr. St. Louis was set up for a comfortable retirement. The St. Louises paid off their home in The Glebe and their vacation home in Morin-Heights. Dr. St. Louis continued to owe a mortgage on her commercial building on Bank Street.

Through diligent savings and by drawing a salary and dividends from the Professional Corp. as needed, Dr. St. Louis managed to save $500,000 in personally held open investments and another $1,000,000 in investments within her Professional Corp. Dr. St. Louis had also accumulated $800,000 in her IPP. Upon the sale of the practice, the IPP would no longer be funded. Paul would provide various options for drawing an income from these savings, such as transferring to a Life Income Fund (LIF) or purchasing a life annuity.

> *Take care of your financial health the same way you advise patients to take care of their physical health—with the appropriate professionals at their side.*

With her practice valued at $1,000,000, Dr. St. Louis' net worth was in the neighbourhood of $5 million. They were fortunate to also expect Professor St. Louis' pension from the university. If she'd wanted to, she could have walked away and not looked back, but a couple of years prior, she had talked with Paul about the need for an exit strategy. The sale of her business would be the largest transaction of her professional career. Paul left it up to Dr. St. Louis to set the timeline, and she decided that it was time to execute that strategy.

Chapter 21: The exit strategy

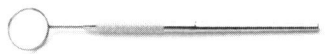

Twelve years ago, Dr. St. Louis had purchased a commercially zoned property on Bank Street and invested heavily in keeping it a well-appointed and immaculate home to her practice. As she approached retirement and planned her exit strategy, she was seeking both a sale of her practice and a more conventional real estate deal. Paul helped her set up a separate corporation for its ownership. She had a few available options. For example, she could have considered holding on to the property and leasing it to the dentist who purchased her practice and the property. It could then serve as a source of income for the St. Louises in their retirement.

This wasn't Dr. St. Louis' first choice. She and her husband were seeking a simple and unfettered retirement. She had worked hard for many years and didn't want a second career as a property manager; she wanted life to be less complicated. The sale of the property was just another factor that complicated negotiations and all part of the overall sale of her practice.

Dr. St. Louis wasn't facing a steep learning curve on the sale of her practice; she'd discussed this with Paul on many occasions and read all the quarterly newsletters issued by the Leighton team over the years. The information in the newsletters provided her with valuable tips and advice that made her as well-versed as any of her peers in matters of tax issues and financial planning. It was one of the reasons she was flagged by her colleagues at events like the annual conference—they were eager to solicit her opinion about their own plans.

> *The metrics for valuations of practices vary widely. Generally, 70 to 100 percent of a year's gross income represents a fair price for both the buyer and vendor, but that's only a starting point.*

She fully understood the numbers and issues involved in the sale of her practice, and had studied the market for dental practices. In the last few years, she'd tried to stay on top of sales of practices in Eastern Ontario, and she'd also perused websites dedicated to the sales of practices. Paul and the Leighton team were doing their part and had referred the valuation of Dr. St. Louis' practice to a third-party broker and evaluator, which was standard practice.

The metrics for valuations of practices varied widely. Generally, 70 to 100 percent of a year's gross income represented a fair price for both the buyer and vendor, but that was only a starting point, and other things had to be considered. In recent years,

SECTION III: DR. ST. LOUIS' EXIT STRATEGY

Dr. St. Louis had gradually improved her practice's efficiency. The practice management consultant referred by the Leighton team had coached her staff to become more effective in their roles, combined with Dr. St. Louis' efforts to maintain reasonable but fair compensation. For the last financial year, expenses represented only 50 percent of gross income before compensation to herself or her family. With an excellent net income, the practice became even more attractive for the purchaser, and Dr. St. Louis was in a better position to command closer to 100 percent of annual gross income in the sale.

> *With an excellent net income, the practice becomes even more attractive for the purchaser, placing the vendor in a better position to command closer to 100 percent of annual gross income in the sale.*

She also understood the dynamics of the market. "It's a seller's market," Paul had told her. When she'd first floated the idea of retirement and the sale of her practice, she'd fielded a couple of serious bids and taken on potential buyers as associates. Those bids fell short of Dr. St. Louis' targets, and, more importantly, she felt the timing wasn't quite right. As she'd frequently explained to her husband during previous attempts to sell her practice, it was "big enough not to do if it were only *almost* right." There was also a point of pride and emotional investment for Dr. St. Louis—she'd built her practice from the ground up, and she believed that any sort of discount for expedience would devalue her hard work.

When Dr. Parry first approached Dr. St. Louis about becoming her associate, he gently broached the subject of purchasing the practice one day. Dr. St. Louis was candid with Dr. Parry about the fact that the subject had been raised by other young dentists who'd previously worked as her associates. On those other occasions, it had come down to timing and fit—Dr. St. Louis felt it was either too soon for her to step aside, or she wasn't quite comfortable with the associates who'd expressed interest in her practice. After those disappointments, Dr. St. Louis vowed she would only take on another associate if she were confident that the associate would eventually take over her practice.

It wasn't long, however, before Dr. St. Louis began to have a good feeling about Dr. Parry. Those positive feelings proved prescient. Dr. Parry went on to be a pleasure to work with and proved to be of outstanding character.

Chapter 22: The defining issue: a share- or asset-based sale

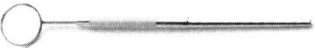

Many years ago, Dr. St. Louis had added her adult children as non-voting shareholders to her Professional Corporation. This had been done for two reasons: to allow dividends to be shared with her children while in low tax brackets, and to allow future capital gains to be taxed in their names. Over the past few years, two of the St. Louises' children had gone on to their own successful professional careers, so the dividends paid to them were reduced

"

Adding adult children as non-voting shareholders to a Professional Corporation allows dividends to be shared with them while in low tax brackets and allows future capital gains to be taxed in their names.

"

149

and funds that had been previously directed to them were folded into retirement plans. Dr. St. Louis had accumulated $1 million in investments within her company from these savings. However, there were still tax-planning benefits to maintaining the children as shareholders upon the eventual sale of her practice.

Her husband, Professor St. Louis, wasn't among the family members named as shareholders. It wasn't an oversight. It simply reflected that with more than a quarter-century of tenure as a university academic, and as associate dean in his faculty, Professor St. Louis drew a healthy salary from the school. In fact, Professor St. Louis' income was high enough that had any dividend been paid to him, it would have been taxed at the highest marginal rate. In addition, corporate attribution issues might have arisen as corporate savings started accumulating, resulting in less-than-desirable tax consequences.

"

The implications for the vendor and the buyer are quite dramatic, depending on whether it's a share or asset sale.

"

An independent valuation placed the practice at $1 million. Also, with $1 million of investment assets within the corporation the value of the company shares totalled $2 million. Like other well-established dentists in similar positions, Dr. St. Louis needed to negotiate the price and structure of the practice sale. The implications for the vendor and the buyer were quite dramatic, depending on whether it would be a share or asset sale.

The Leighton team advised Dr. St. Louis that there were special rules to follow if she wished to sell the shares tax-free. To qualify for the capital gains exemption, she would need to "purify" her company by removing $1 million of investments from the corporation (eventually, the withdrawal of these funds would be taxable anyway). The corporate-owned life insurance policy would also need to be transferred out, but given the nature of the policy, there would be little tax impact. With multiple shareholders, it would be possible to shelter the remaining $1 million attributed to the dental practice from any tax.

The Leighton team prepared a comparison spreadsheet so that the St. Louises could clearly see the impact of both approaches. The team's tax accountant calculated what each approach meant in terms of personal and corporate taxes. The complex calculations involved a thorough review of the advantages and disadvantages of using the capital gains exemption.

"

A share sale means that the proceeds flow directly to the vendor and his or her children. By utilizing the capital gains exemption, they avoid any of the tax.

"

Dr. St. Louis wanted to sell the shares in her practice to Dr. Parry because it had the lowest tax impact to her. A share sale meant that the proceeds would flow directly to Dr. St. Louis and her children. By utilizing the capital gains exemption, Dr. St. Louis and her children avoided any of the tax. Dr. St. Louis preferred not to sell the assets such as goodwill, leaseholds, and dental equipment; otherwise, the total taxes payable would be in the range of $237,000.

On the other hand, Dr. Parry preferred to purchase assets for the tax advantages available to him. An asset sale would allow him to amortize the depreciation of assets for tax purposes. The bulk of savings from amortization would be accrued during the first five years after the sale, in the range of $50,000. Dr. Parry preferred not to purchase shares because it offered him no immediate tax advantages.

"

An asset sale allows the buyer to amortize the depreciation of assets for tax purposes, whereas a share sale offers the buyer no tax relief.

"

Regardless of which method of sale occurred, both parties faced tax implications ranging from $50,000 to $237,000. As Paul saw it, however, this now represented wiggle room for when the actual negotiations of the sale began.

Chapter 23: The final stretch

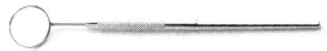

It was now time for Dr. St. Louis to enter into serious negotiations about the purchase of her practice, and her lawyer was exchanging e-mails with Dr. Parry's lawyer about the final arrangements.

In the days and weeks leading up to the final negotiations, Dr. St. Louis and Paul Leighton had discussed the strategy and the impact on her retirement. Paul had also reviewed all the numbers with her and coached her on the position she would take once negotiations began.

"You've done everything right in the management of your finances throughout your career, but this is the last piece of the puzzle," he'd reminded her. "This is the single largest transaction you'll make, and it can play a huge role in hitting the net worth that you targeted for retirement."

Dr. St. Louis had listened intently and nodded. "Paul, I appreciate what you've done for me, and I'm glad to have a chance to talk about a few matters first," she'd said. "I do want to sell this practice, and I'm not quite prepared to go to the wall with this deal. I understand Trevor's desire to push for favourable terms, but I'm not willing to do a deal at any cost. There is a point where I'd walk away."

> "
>
> *Selling a practice is the single largest transaction you'll make, and it can play a huge role in hitting the net worth that you've targeted for retirement.*
>
> "

As Paul had worked out in detail, Dr. Parry would lose tax benefits on a share sale but it would have tax advantages for Dr. St. Louis. A compromise would need to be made. Paul had reviewed more complex deals in the past—such as the sale of a half-share of a practice, effectively making a wholly owned practice into a partnership. This wasn't an approach Paul usually recommended. He recognized the efficiency that a partnership could enjoy, such as the sharing of common overhead expenses such as rent or staff, but he preferred the autonomy of a single practice.

Dr. St. Louis also hadn't wanted to pursue a partnership.

"I've always envisioned a clean break," she'd said. "And taking my equity out of the sale would put me over my target for $3 million in investable assets. I'll exceed my retirement goal."

There would be other issues on the table in the negotiations, but the largest would be the commercial property that housed the practice. At first, Dr. St. Louis had preferred to sell the property; it had a list value of $550,000.

This could have been a difficult issue. Dr. Parry would have had to arrange financing to buy the property, and he had already been working with his bank on the 100 percent financing of the purchase of the practice. It would have been unfortunate and, moreover, inconvenient for Dr. St. Louis to negotiate favourable terms on the purchase of her practice only to see the deal fall through because of the commercial property.

> *The sale of a half-share of a practice effectively makes a wholly owned practice into a partnership.*

Paul had reminded her that she had considerable net equity in the property, in terms of her net worth, so it didn't particularly matter if she sold the property immediately or stayed on as landlord. He'd asked the Leighton team's commercial real estate expert to give Dr. St. Louis an idea of the leasing revenues that similar properties were generating in Ottawa. This would have made her more than comfortable with the idea of holding on to it for a while if this meant keeping the negotiations moving forward.

After reviewing the numbers, Dr. St. Louis had said, "The equity will still be working for me with the rental revenue contributing toward my retirement income. And there's a good chance that my equity will increase if the commercial real estate market heats up at all."

When negotiations had begun, Dr. St. Louis had told her lawyer that she was open to leasing the property to Dr. Parry and that she didn't want the terms of the lease to hold up negotiations. "We can base the monthly rental amount on the amount paid out for a just-signed lease in an adjacent building," she'd explained.

Dr. Parry had presented his first choice regarding the property: leasing the property from Dr. St. Louis with the idea that, down the line, he might buy it from her. They'd agreed to a five-year term plus another five-year renewal option, with the opportunity to purchase the building at fair market value at the end of the initial five-year term.

The first offer from Dr. Parry had given Dr. St. Louis something to work with: $900,000 for the shares in practice. It was the valuation of the practice, less $100,000. Clearly Dr. Parry had been in earnest when he'd said that he was prepared to buy the practice as assets for $1 million.

The two sides had gone back and forth on the numbers, and Dr. St. Louis now finally agreed to a third counteroffer of $950,000. She was going to net the full amount tax-free from the sale of the shares of her practice. It was a done deal.

"Congratulations," Paul said when Dr. St. Louis called to inform him that the deal had closed successfully.

Dr. St. Louis felt safe to confide in Paul. "I feel an immense sense of relief that this is over."

"Sorry to break it to you, but it's not quite over yet," Paul said. "We have to prepare the filings for our tax team, and we'll have to figure out what will be the best possible place to park the proceeds from the sale, and any investment positions that you might want to pursue going forward."

Dr. St. Louis sighed.

"Don't worry," Paul said. "It's just like signing a golf card at the end of the best round of your life. You've put yourself in a position to enjoy yourself comfortably for the rest of your life."

SECTION III: DR. ST. LOUIS' EXIT STRATEGY

The rest of her life. Dr. St. Louis couldn't wait to get started.

"

Put yourself in a position to enjoy yourself comfortably for the rest of your life.

"

Chapter 24: Celebrating with friends

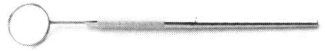

Over the eighteen months Dr. Parry had spent as an associate in Dr. St. Louis' practice, he'd brought in a steady stream of patients and increased his own workload. Dr. St. Louis' husband had taken on a lighter load of classroom hours, and she'd scaled back her workload so that she no longer worked Monday afternoons and Fridays. So even though the annual ODA conference started on a Thursday, Dr. St. Louis and her husband came into Toronto the previous Monday night so they could take in a play and a musical. Tuesday night, she and her husband would dine at some lovely restaurant downtown and then escape to the vibrant, fun world of the theatre for a few hours. Dr. St. Louis was quite excited.

A couple of weeks before, when Dr. St. Louis reserved tickets for their flight and hotel room, she'd sent an e-mail to Dr. Malhotra asking if he and Anita could come to Toronto on Wednesday night to go out to dinner. Dr. Malhotra accepted the invitation, but suggested that Dr. Bekker and his wife join them as well. Dr. St. Louis was surprised by Dr. Malhotra's suggestion—she hadn't been aware that he'd been in contact with Dr. Bekker, other than their chance meetings at the once-a-year ODA conference.

The more the merrier, Dr. St. Louis wrote back.

Allow me to pick out a spot—Anita and I have a favourite place and we know you'll be delighted with it, Dr. Malhotra said in his next e-mail. *I'll contact Dennis as well.*

Dr. Malhotra sent an e-mail to Dr. Bekker to ask if he and his wife would be available for dinner that Wednesday. *We'd be delighted,* Dr. Bekker responded. *Anything that keeps us from skiing!* The Bekkers hadn't quite given up on skiing, but they were spending more time in front of the fireplace at their cottage than on chairlifts. They had planned to stay home that evening because their daughters would be coming home from school, and they quite honestly missed them and wanted to spend time catching up and hearing about finals and summer plans. A few hours would be fine, they reasoned. It would give the girls a chance to settle in without having their parents hovering over them, at least not right away.

The Bekkers could also make an occasion of the night out—in years past, they'd dined out frequently. Now, though, they were eating in more often. Mrs. Bekker figured it was better for their waistlines, and they found that they enjoyed eating a gourmet meal at home for a change. Dr. Bekker had even e-mailed Dr. Malhotra requesting a few simple recipes that he could make. And he was proud to say he could now make crepes filled with cheese and ham. It delighted Mrs. Bekker to no end.

The three couples met that Wednesday night at a popular downtown restaurant suggested by Dr. Malhotra. He'd heard rave reviews about the menu—so much so that he planned to come back Saturday after the conference. He didn't want to simply sample the fare; he was planning to try his hand at recreating the dishes he liked best at home.

The evening air was warm and fragrant, as winter was on its way out and spring was at its heels. As with the change in seasons, so too were there changes in the lives of all three dentists. It seemed it was an evening for announcements. Dr. Malhotra went first.

"Anita and I have some news to share about our wedding. We've set a date for this August, and you're all invited!" he said.

"That's fantastic!" said Mrs. Bekker. "Anita, you'll make a lovely bride."

"We're planning to bring over a few of my relatives from Delhi. It's not official—just tentative plans—but we're looking at going to Italy and France for our honeymoon."

"There's no shortage of good food there!" Dr. Bekker said. "I'm sure you won't be doing all the cooking. Congratulations, Arjun and Anita. That's good news."

"That's not all," Anita interjected.

All eyes at the table turned to Dr. Malhotra again.

"We've also purchased a house in London. It's in a newer area and is being built for us. We get to pick our upgrades this week," he said.

The planning set in place a couple of years before by Paul Leighton and his associates was bearing fruit. Dr. Malhotra held off on sharing one other piece of news simply because airing it seemed premature—he was in the final stages of buying Dr. Tarber's practice in London. He and Anita had been at Paul Leighton's office earlier that week to review the final valuation report of Dr. Tarber's practice and to discuss bank financing of the purchase.

Dr. Malhotra and Anita had also consulted with the Leighton team's tax expert on establishing a dental hygiene corporation with Anita as the main shareholder. A hygiene corporation would offer additional tax planning opportunities as they continued to grow the practice together. Dr. Malhotra was confident that he'd own the practice within a couple of months, but discussing it now would feel like tempting fate.

"Well, since we seem to be sharing news, I have some as well," Dr. St. Louis said, looking at the colleagues who'd become friends over the years. "My husband and I have been planning our retirements for some time," she said, smiling. "I've completed a deal and sold my practice! You might remember my associate, Dr. Parry, from last year's conference..."

Both Dr. Malhotra and Dr. Bekker did.

"Dr. Parry purchased my practice last month," she told them. "All the planning prior to the sale certainly paid off, and I'm very pleased and relieved by the outcome," she confided. "Now, my husband and I look forward to enjoying our retirement and travelling more."

"Congratulations, Adeline, we're very happy for you!" Dr. Malhotra said.

"That's good news," said Dr. Bekker, raising his glass. "Here's to retirement and finally reaping what you sow. Good for you, Adeline. Cheers!" he said and then took a hearty swallow of his brandy.

Everyone raised their glasses to share a toast, but Dr. St. Louis stopped them all. "Wait a minute, here we are toasting our good fortune, but Dennis, do you have anything to add to the toast? Some good news on your part?"

"We went skiing, and I didn't fall," Mrs. Bekker said.

That brought laughter around the entire table.

"Very funny, Trish. What she *meant* to say is that our son is engaged," Dr. Bekker said.

"And our daughters aren't," Mrs. Bekker said, letting out a sigh of relief.

"Now we can have a toast to good fortune for all of us. Cheers, to new friends and bright futures," said Dr. St. Louis. Everyone raised their glasses in agreement.

Dr. Adeline St. Louis, DMD

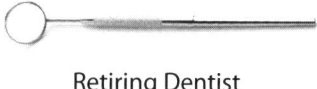

Retiring Dentist

- Age 60

- Graduated 33 years ago from the The Faculty of Dentistry, McGill University

- Dental practice located in Ottawa

- Client of Leighton team for well over 15 years.

Dr. St. Louis had been served well for many years by having a cohesive financial plan prepared and monitered by the Leighton Team. Now it was time to move to the final phase of that plan: the exit strategy. This is what it looked like.

Goals

- Practice sale and transition, share sale vs. asset sale decision
- Sale of dental building now or later
- Achieve retirement goal of $180,000 per year for desired lifestyle, with $120,000 coming from savings and $60,000 from Professor St. Louis' pension
- Comprehensive estate plan

Cash Flow

INCOME

Salary to Dr. St. Louis	$125,000
Salary to Professor St. Louis	$135,000
Personal Tax & CPP	($80,000)
Net cash flow	**$180,000**

LIFESTYLE EXPENSES

Home and vacation property	$50,000
Food and other household expenses	$24,000
Automobile expenses	$18,000
Personal discretionary spending	$48,000
Disability and Critical Illness insurance	$10,000
Savings/Buffer	$30,000
Total annual spending	**$180,000**

Net Worth

ASSETS

Home	$900,000
Vacation Property	$500,000
Vehicles	$50,000
Individual Pension Plan (IPP)	$800,000
Tax-Free Savings Account (TFSA)	$30,000
Open Investments (personal)	$500,000
Open Investments (Professional Corporation)	$1,000,000
Dental Practice (prior to sale)	$1,000,000
Dental Building	$550,000
	$5,330,000

LIABILITIES

Commercial Property	$250,000
Tax debts on sale of shares & investments	$326,000
	$576,000

NET WORTH   **$4,754,000**

Practice Sale: a share or asset-based sale

Dr. St. Louis, the vendor, preferred to sell shares to take advantage of the $750,000 Capital Gains Exemption. This exemption is available to Dr. St. Louis and each of her children, so entire $1M practice value easily sheltered from tax.

Dr. Parry, the buyer, preferred to purchase assets of the practice (e.g. goodwill, leaseholds, equipment) as it would allow him to amortize the assets for tax savings.

This calculation is based on a practice valuation of $1,000,000.

SALE OF SHARES

Purification of company required	$1,000,000
(redeem investments, assume FMV equals ACB)	
Personal Tax on Dividends @ 32.6%	($326,000)
Net after withdrawal of investments	$674,000
Proceeds of Share Sale	$1,000,000
(tax-free due to Capital Gains Exemption)	
Net Cash Flow after all taxes	**$1,674,000**

Practice Sale: a share or asset-based sale (continued)

SALE OF ASSETS

Goodwill		$800,000
Assets (equipment, leaseholds)		$200,000
Proceeds of sale before tax		$1,000,000
Goodwill	$800,000	
Taxable Portion (@ 50%)	$400,000	
Tax on Goodwill (@15.5%)	($62,000)	
Corporate tax		($62,000)
Net proceeds after tax		$938,000
Investment Assets		$1,000,000
Withdrawal of investments and after-tax profits from corporation		$1,938,000
Tax-free portion of goodwill @ 50% (taken through Capital Dividend Account)		($400,000)
Remainder distributed as dividend to Dr. St. Louis		$1,538,000
Personal tax on dividend @ 32.6%		($501,000)
Cash flow after tax on dividend		$1,037,000
Tax-free portion of goodwill		$400,000
Net Cash Flow after all taxes		**$1,437,000**
NET SAVINGS (selling shares instead of assets)		**$237,000**

These calculations are based on the initial practice valuation of $1,000,000.
However, after negotiations, the shares of the practice were sold for $950,000.

Retirement Planning

The St. Louises' desired retirement lifestyle demanded an income of $180,000 per year, derived from the following sources:

Individual Pension Plan (IPP)	$800,000
TFSA	$30,000
Open Investments	$500,000
Proceeds of Sale (shares)	$1,674,000
	$3,004,000
Withdrawal from Investments (@ 4%)	$120,000
Professor St. Louis' pension	$60,000
Annual retirement income	**$180,000**

Estate Plan

- Use of primary and secondary wills to avoid probate fees on shares of the Professional Corporation, saving up to 1.5% ($30,000)
- Use of testamentary trusts for the benefit of the children, with potential for tax reduction on investment income, and extra level of security in the event a child finds themselves in a troubled marriage
- Use of permanent life insurance to offset tax payable by the estate

Results

- Share sale was negotiated with a reduced price of $950,000 to factor lack of tax saving opportunity for Dr. Parry and allowing $750,000 tax-free capital gains exemption to Dr. St. Louis with net savings of $237,000.

- Building was not sold, lease terms were negotiated (5 years plus 5 years), with option for Dr. Parry to purchase at anytime at fair market value

- With prudent low-cost-index-type investment strategies and a well-diversified portfolio, investing, and sale of dental practice, Dr. St. Louis' target asset level ($3,004,000) accomplished

- Investment portfolio adjusted to reflect retirement and cash flow needs of $120,000 annually.

- Established a comprehensive estate plan through use of secondary wills, testamentary trusts, and life insurance, saving significant taxes.

Epilogue

Dr. Malhotra: Five-year profile

Dr. Malhotra moved into his new home six weeks after the annual association conference. Later that year, Dr. Malhotra and Anita's wedding was a rousing success. The dividends paid out to his parents helped to underwrite the expenses incurred by relatives who travelled from Delhi for the ceremony. In five years, their new $500,000 home was paid off.

Dr. Malhotra negotiated the purchase of a practice in London for $750,000, and it was growing. The Leighton team helped him arrange 100-percent financing for the purchase.

For the last year prior to the transition, Dr. Malhotra worked as an associate in that practice. His wife, Anita, started working there as a full-time hygienist after the purchase. His incorporation allowed him to pay off his student loan and contribute to a retirement savings plan set up by the Leighton team.

Dr. Bekker: Five-year profile

The Bekkers' finances stabilized, their debts were paid down ten years sooner than they would have been, and their cash flow improved significantly.

Dr. Bekker managed to increase his billings by 10 percent, passing the $1-million mark, while reducing the ratio of expenses to profit to his targeted 50:50.

Dividends from Dr. Bekker's incorporated practice were able to underwrite his son's and twin daughters' college educations. The improved profitability allowed the Bekkers to invest savings from the corporation into a corporate investment and Individual Pension Plans, and they planned to increase those contributions once their children completed graduation. Using low-cost index–type investment strategies and a well-diversified portfolio, their needs were addressed. The Bekkers set up new life, disability, and critical illness insurance policies.

Dr. St. Louis: Five-year profile

After the transfer of the practice to Dr. Parry, Dr. St. Louis retired as planned. Professor St. Louis taught part-time for a year and went on a sabbatical year, during which he planned to write another book.

The St. Louises travelled extensively during this sabbatical year. With comprehensive and well-planned strategies from having worked with the Leighton team for over fifteen years, the St. Louises improved their cash flow, reduced their taxes, and achieved their net worth targets, aligning Dr. St. Louis' practice with their lives to enjoy a comfortable retirement, drawing $120,000 annually from their investments.

About the Authors

MIKE LAKHANI, B.Comm, F.C.C.A., C.G.A., CFP, R.F.P.

One of Assante Wealth Management's top advisors, Mike leads Assante's largest branch network with client assets under administration exceeding $1.6 billion. Prior to joining Assante, Mike was the president and founding member of Investment and Tax Counsel Corp. Having worked in the business since 1987, Mike brings expertise in tax planning, accounting, and personal financial planning to dental clients. Mike manages a "Family Office," a one-stop center for dentists, aligning clients' dental practices with their personal lives. With access under one roof to expert seasoned professionals for tax planning, accounting, cash management, practice issues, retirement planning, structured portfolios, estate planning and insurance, each client's unique needs are efficiently implemented. Mike is the author of the newsletter *Tax Matters for Dentists*, together with his partners, Stive Farronato and Chris Molloy.

With an ongoing goal to be among the best in an industry where knowledge and keeping up to date with the latest changes is critical, Mike holds several professional designations, including Fellow of the Association of Chartered Certified Accountants, Certified General Accountant, Chartered Financial Planner, and Registered Financial Planner. Mike believes in combining professional dedication and personal commitment to offer creative planning in the context of a personal and caring relationship.

STIVE FARRONATO, CA, CFP
A Chartered Accountant and financial planning advisor, Stive specializes in providing advanced tax planning strategies for the dental professional. Stive graduated from the University of Toronto in 1989. After articling for two years, he received the Chartered Accountant (CA) designation in 1992 and his Certified Financial Planning (CFP) designation in 1998. Previously, Stive worked in public practice from 1989 to 1993 and with the Canada Revenue Agency from 1993 to 1995. Stive has been part of Mike Lakhani's team at Assante Wealth Management since 1995. He is a co-author of *Tax Matters for Dentists*.

CHRIS MOLLOY, B.A.Sc., CFP
A financial planning advisor with Assante Wealth Management Ltd. and co-author of *Tax Matters for Dentists*, Chris has over fifteen years of experience advising clients on tax, investment, and estate planning strategies to achieve their financial goals. Chris believes in helping clients make informed choices and takes great pride in developing comprehensive financial plans for dentists.

Prior to joining Assante, Chris worked as a financial advisor with one of Canada's largest life insurance companies. Chris has been part of Mike Lakhani's team since 1996.